Sexual strategies

For Pleasure and Safety

The Institute for Advanced Study of Human Sexuality

Ted McIlvenna, M. Div., Ph.D., A.C.S., and
Roe Gallo, Ph.D., M.P.H., A.C.S., co-editors

Clark Taylor, Ph.D., Ed.D., M.P.H.,
Special Research Consultant

Specific Press
San Francisco

Published by Specific Press
1523 Franklin St.
San Francisco CA 94109

Cover design by Greg Pless

Cover Photo: Corbis.com

Printed in the United States of America on acid-free paper

Library of Congress Cataloging-in-Publication Data
Sexual Strategies for Pleasure and Safety /
    editors, Ted McIlvenna, Roe Gallo
    "To empower the reader to create a pleasurable and safer
    sex life." - Intro.
    Includes index.

ISBN 0-930846-25-7

DEDICATION

This book is dedicated to Clark Taylor, Ph.D., Ed.D, M.P.H. Dr. Taylor made a life long commitment to the study of Human Sexuality and HIV/AIDS. His contributions to this field of Human Sexuality, both as a researcher and a teacher, are far too extensive to list here.

ABOUT THE EDITORS

Ted McIlvenna is the founder and president of the Institute for Advanced Study of Human Sexuality. He is a former athlete, an accomplished musician, a theologian, an academician and a true social and educational designer. Dr. McIlvenna is the author of 16 books and the producer of 122 sex education films and videos. He is also the trustee of the world's largest erotology collection. Dr. McIlvenna is a sexologist committed to the integration of sexology with other academic disciplines. He is a strong advocate for personal and sexual rights and the preservation of our sexual heritage.

Contact information: www.iashs.edu

Roe Gallo is an author, researcher, professional speaker and sexologist. She earned her Masters degree from San Francisco State University in Health Communication and her Ph.D. and M.P.H. from the Institute for Advanced Study of Human Sexuality. Dr. Gallo has lead lectures and workshops and brings with her nearly 20 years of health education experience. She is currently an adjunct professor at San Francisco State University. Her published works include: Body Ecology, Perfect Body the Raw Truth and Perfect Body Beyond the Illusion.

Contact information: www. roegallo.com

CONTENTS

PREFACE

*S*exual Strategies for Pleasure and Safety is a carefully devised plan of action to enjoy sex and not get STD's.

Throughout this book, I use the more popular acronym STD when referring to sexually transmitted disease and infection, including HIV/AIDS.

Fear is not the answer for prevention! The incidences of STD's have increased over the years, with each year bringing more cases and more deaths. The fear has also increased and yet people are still getting infected.

The campaign for sexual abstinence is not the answer! Abstinence is a choice and should not take the place of safer sex education. The dramatic increase in STD's has shown itself in the heterosexual community and especially among young adults and children. In 2001, the CDC reported an increase in STD's and that the highest incidence was in the 10 - 24 year old age group. This is a substantial increase in younger teenagers.

Sexual rights and sexual responsibility equal sexual health and pleasure! You have a natural right to sexual freedom and pleasure and with that right brings the responsibly for your own sexual health and pleasure. It is up to you, as an individual, to take care of yourself. You cannot rely on, or expect, anyone else to protect you! This includes friends, family, lovers, government, medicine.

Knowledge and strategies are the answer! Knowledge of STD's, risk and prevention and concrete strategies to stay sexually healthy and create sexual pleasure.

Roe Gallo, Ph.D., M.P.H., A.C.S

INTRODUCTION

*I*n *Sexual Strategies for Pleasure and Safety,* the objective is to enjoy sex and not get STD's. **The main focus of the book is to empower the reader to create a pleasurable and safer sex life.** The focus is on the prevention for all STD's and not just HIV/AIDS, because if you expose yourself to any STD, you will be exposing yourself to all STD's, including HIV/AIDS.

The information in this book will help you to:

1. Keep free of STD's.
2. Manage any STD's you may have.
3. Have sex without fear.
4. Enjoy your sexuality alone and with others.
5. Be responsible for your sexuality.
6. Be responsible for your health and safety.
7. Learn about yourself and your body
8. Make informed choices and decisions about your sexual lifestyle.
9. Know the latest available and sex positive information about the cause, risk and prevention of STD's.
10. Know safe sex techniques that, as much as possible, do not detract from and possibly enhance, the pleasure and meaning of sexuality.
11. Know practical alternatives and suggestions.
12. Know an approach to STD's that is in accord with basic human sexual rights.

Basic human rights must be built around freedom of choice. There can be no freedom, if there is no choice. The number one weapon is education and education must include basic sexual rights.

These Basic Sexual Rights were adopted by the faculty of the Institute for Advanced Study of Human Sexuality in 1981 and are still serving the faculty and student body as they face the challenges of the 21st Century.

The Basic Sexual Rights are:

1. The freedom of any sexual thought, fantasy or desire.
2. The right to sexual entertainment, freely available in the marketplace, including sexually explicit materials dealing with the full range of sexual behavior.
3. The right not to be exposed to sexual material or behavior.
4. The right to sexual self-determination.
5. The right to seek out and engage in consensual sexual activity.
6. The right to engage in sexual acts or activities of any kind whatsoever, providing they do not involve nonconsensual acts, violence, constraint, coercion or fraud.
7. The right to be free of persecution, condemnation, discrimination, or societal intervention in private sexual behavior.
8. The recognition by society that every person, partnered or unpartnered, has the right to the pursuit of a satisfying consensual sociosexual life free from political, legal or religious interference and that there need to be mechanisms in society where the opportunities of sociosexual activities are available to the following: disabled persons; chronically ill persons; those incarcerated in prisons, hospitals or institutions; those disadvantaged because of age, lack of physical attractiveness, or lack of social skills; the poor and the lonely.
9. The basic right of all persons who are sexually dysfunctional to have available nonjudgmental sexual health care.
10. The right to control conception.

CHAPTER ONE: SEX WITHOUT FEAR

*S*exual Strategies for Pleasure and Safety is a no nonsense book on how to have pleasurable and fulfilling sex while protecting yourself from sexually transmitted diseases (STD's) and sexually transmitted infections (STI's), including HIV/AIDS. For the purpose of simplicity, "STD's" will be used when referring to sexually transmitted diseases and infections, including HIV/AIDS. Although STI's is used in most of the medical literature, STD's is the popular and most common term.

This book is designed to provide the facts so that you can make informed decisions about what you want, and don't want, sexually. Following this guide helps put *you* in control of your sex life, your sexual health and your pleasure.

Gratifying sexual expression is life enhancing and trying to stop people from being sexual is futile. The position of this book is not to stop you from having sex but to show you how to the reduce risk of getting STD's.

Sex is a natural and healthy part of life. Cultural, religious and social taboos about sex may make it difficult to get correct information about safety. You have the right to your sexuality. You have a right to pleasure. You have a right to accurate information about how to protect yourself from becoming infected.

Knowledge Is Power

Accurate information will help you determine your level of risk and better decide what course of action you need to take to feel safer and enjoy sex.

Again, the objective of this book is to enjoy sex and not get STD's. The main focus of the book is to empower the reader to approach safer sex with total candor within the context of what people actually do sexually. STD's and unwanted pregnancies cannot be prevented unless you improve your understanding of all sexual behavior and develop adequate sexual risk reduction strategies. This is difficult, if not impossible, to accomplish with sex negative attitudes. A first step to changing those attitudes and preparing for safer and more pleasurable sex is to allow yourself to get over sexual embarrassment, prudery and objections to the sexual practices of those different from you.

You cannot rely on sexual denial or abstinence-only programs to help reduce the risk of STD's and unwanted pregnancies. These programs have been shown, throughout history, to increase the incidents of STD's. People will have sex, in committed relationships or not, and ignorance of STD's will continue to create more disease, and in the case of HIV – death. Education is the solution! You need accurate information about disease, risk and prevention. You also need to learn ways to make high-risk activities less risky without sacrificing enjoyment and without increasing fear.

In order to stay healthy it is important for you to:
- Know about STD's
- Determine your level of risk
- Understand how to protect yourself
- Get tested regularly

This Book is for Everyone

Sexual Strategies for Pleasure and Safety is both a general reference book on the sexual aspects of STD prevention and a "how to" book for people who want to create a safer, healthier and more pleasurable sexual lifestyle.

Sexual Strategies for Pleasure and Safety will empower you with skills to:

- Recognize the signs and symptoms of all STD's and the risks involved.
- Protect yourself against all STD's.
- Develop a sex positive attitude
- Make informed choices about what you want and don't want sexually
- Communicate with your partner(s).
- Enrich and enjoy sex with yourself and/or your partner(s)

Sexual Strategies for Pleasure and Safety adheres to the following principles:

- Everyone has a right to a good sex life.
- Sex can, and should, be the subject of serious, open and nonjudgmental discussion.
- To facilitate healthy sexual choices, people need sexual knowledge, scientific facts and the ability to discuss sexual issues.
- Each individual is responsible for determining his or her own level of risk, comfort and pleasure.
- Each individual has the ability to create a satisfying safer sex lifestyle.
- No one should dictate your sexual activity and disease prevention. NO ONE!!! Not partners! Not law or government! Sexuality is the most individualistic part of a person's life and has never been successfully legislated or controlled by force or coercion.

CHAPTER TWO: STD's

Symptoms are not always present, therefore, you may be infected and not know it!

STD's can be transmitted when infected body fluids, (semen, vaginal discharge, blood (includes menstrual blood), ulcerations), contact mucosal surfaces (example, the male urethra, the vagina or cervix, the mouth, open wounds) and, in the case of genital herpes, syphilis and HPV, the skin.

When people first learn about STD's, they often react in a variety of ways depending on the degree to which they personalize the risk. These include indifference, shock, fear, denial, shame, anger, helplessness, numbness, depression, self-righteousness, indignation, hostility and/or vindictiveness. While these feelings are natural, they do not stop STD transmission. Some people experience a loss of sexual interest; others have increased sexual activity. Be assured that responsible sex can be erotic and satisfying. In fact, if safer sex is part of negotiations for sociosexual activity, it can actually increase sexual intimacy.

There are many STD's, however the following are the most serious and common ones:
- Human immunodeficiency virus (HIV)
- Gonorrhea
- Chlamydia
- Trichomoniasis (Trich)
- Genital herpes
- Syphilis
- Human papillomavirus (HPV)

HIV/AIDS

Human immunodeficiency virus (HIV) destroys the immune system and leaves it susceptible for infection with bacteria and other viruses. When a person's immune system can no longer protect them, they are diagnosed with Aquired Immune Deficiency Syndrome (AIDS).

HIV enters the body either as free virus present in body fluids or encapsulated in blood or other cells. Outside the body, HIV cannot live long and is very easy to kill, however, once inside a person's body, the virus attaches to cells and works its way inside. The virus may remain dormant for long periods of time and then, takes over the genetic material of the cell and makes copies of itself, replicating in great numbers (CDC, 2002).

Other Strains of HIV

Powerful treatments can bring the load of native virus in a person's system to undetectable level, because of that you may become re-infected with viral strains that are resistant to HIV drugs. Therefore, if you are infected, you must refrain from having unsafe sex with other people who are also infected. Otherwise, super strains of HIV can occur and increase your susceptibility to other infections.

Cofactors

HIV becomes much more deadly when certain other problems or "cofactors" are present.

Some of these cofactors are:
- A lifestyle that weakens the immune system such as alcohol and drug abuse, chronic stress and malnutrition.

- Pathogens that weaken the immune system, particularly cytomegalovirus (CMV) and Epstein-Barr virus (EBV).
- Common sexually transmitted disease – trichomoniasis, syphilis, herpes and candidiasis (yeast) – create conditions that can greatly facilitate the transmission of HIV. The lesions that these pathogens create appear to be routes of transmission and, in themselves, can become so serious in advanced HIV disease that they can cause death.

How it is transmitted

HIV can be transmitted in many different ways from one person to another.

These are the most common ways of transmission:
- by having unprotected sex (anal, vaginal, or oral) with an HIV-infected person
- by sharing needles or injection equipment with an HIV-infected person
- from HIV-infected women to babies before or during birth, or through breast feeding after birth
- occasionally contaminated blood transfusions

You can also get HIV when instruments contaminated with blood are either not sterilized or disinfected or are used inappropriately between clients. This includes medical, dental, tattoo and/or body piercing. CDC recommends that instruments that are intended to penetrate the skin be used once, then disposed of or thoroughly cleaned and sterilized (CDC, 2002).

Fallacies about Transmission

HIV/AIDS is not transmitted through casual contact such as shaking hands, hugging, social kissing, sneezing, coughing, face-to-face conversation, touching or sitting close to an infected person. Remember, the virus is very fragile outside the body and must travel by way of infected body fluids (semen, vaginal discharge, blood, ulcerations) into the body through mucosal surfaces (e.g., the male urethra, the vagina or cervix, the mouth, open wounds)

Who gets infected?

According to the Center for Disease Control (CDC), AIDS is no longer considered a "gay" related disease; HIV can infect anyone. HIV is transmitted by risky activities, not by sexual orientation. HIV-related illness and death now have the greatest impact on young people and among people of heterosexual orientation.

Also, according to the CDC, AIDS is a leading cause of death among Americans 25 to 44 years-old. In this same age group, AIDS now accounts on average for 1 in every 3 deaths among African-American men and 1 in 5 deaths in African-American women (CDC, 2001).

A study by the National Cancer Institute, confirms a substantial increase in the rate of infection as individuals enter their late teens and early twenties, with infection rates peaking in the mid-to-late twenties (CDC, 2001).

Pregnant Women and HIV

Both partners should be tested before pregnancy occurs. People who test positive might choose not to have children. If you test positive and you are pregnant, your baby could be born HIV positive.

If you are HIV negative and already pregnant, safe sex techniques, with any partner, are especially important. Artificial insemination should come from HIV-negative donors only. Frozen sperm is probably safer than fresh.

Pregnant women can obtain HIV test results in labor! This is important in order to start antiretroviral therapy as soon as possible. Such timely knowledge of the mother's HIV status also provides opportunities for other interventions that reduce transmission, such as elective cesarean section, avoiding artificial rupture of membranes, and avoiding breastfeeding.

According to the Mother Infant Rapid Intervention At Delivery (MIRIAD) study (11/19/01 – 11/1/02) (CDC, 2002), when the OraQuick Rapid HIV-1 Antibody Test was tested at delivery on 1771 pregnant women, 12 HIV-positive mothers identified. Also, there were no false-negative and no false-positive tests.

Symptoms

People are most infectious at the beginning of the disease when they are least likely to show symptoms.

Within a couple of weeks or months after infection, a person may experience flu-like symptoms that signal the onset of HIV infection. This is usually followed by a long "latency" or "asymptotic" period during which people feel well and have no signs of disease, however they are infectious. This can last 10 years or more. The Centers for Disease Control and Prevention (CDC) has estimated that one fourth of the approximately 900,000 HIV-infected people in the United States are not aware that they are infected.

If the infection is discovered early and treated with care, the disease free period of infection can be decades.

When the immune system is very weak and the amount of virus very high, a wide range of infections develop, some fatal, and this is the stage called AIDS.

HIV Antibody Testing

When HIV enters the body, it begins to attack certain white blood cells called T4 lymphocyte cells (helper cells) or CD4 cells. The immune system then produces antibodies to fight off the infection. Their presence is used to confirm HIV infection. Most HIV tests look for the presence of HIV antibodies; they do not test for the virus itself.

Some struggle with the issue of testing. This is a very complex decision that depends on many conflicting factors. Many are so equally balanced between wanting to know and being afraid to find out that you need help in making the decision and dealing with the outcome. You must not be afraid to seek help if you are stuck. And remember, early detection of HIV infection can prolong life by making proper medical monitoring and treatment possible.

OraQuick Rapid HIV-1 Antibody Test

This anti-body test, approved in November, 2002, uses only one drop of blood and results are available in 20 minutes.

DNA Polymerase Chain Reaction Tests (DNA PCR)

The DNA PCR tests the body's genetic structure for HIV, the actual infection, not just the antibodies. An infection of HIV may be detected just about 2 weeks of exposure.

DNA PCR is used as a diagnostic test in the window between infection and detection - when antibodies may not be detected in an infected individual. (Vogel, 1999).

Adult Industry Medical Health Care Foundation (AIM) a non-profit organization with services now offered to the general public, uses the DNA PCR test and has done over 15,000 tests over the past four years and has had only 2 false positives and no false negatives. They also confirm each positive result by the standard Western Blot and RNA (viral load test).

AIM has over 40 affiliates nationwide to do DNA PCR testing by mail. Go to the AIM website http://aim-med.org/ and follow the instructions for testing by mail. AIM will fax all the info to the affiliate lab or Doctor's office along with the Doctor's order (the DNA PCR test requires one) and a release for you to sign at the time of the draw. The lab draws blood and sends the specimen overnight by Fed Ex to AIM. You get the results in 2 to 3 days by phone and/or fax.

In the event that you test positive, AIM will make sure that you get the best disclosure counseling through their Affiliates and they will also make sure that your positive result is confirmed by the standard Western Blot test and RNA test (viral load.)

Because AIM is a non-profit organization they can find a free facility for counseling and medications in most all states. You can also call AIM for as much counseling as you need.

Special Risk Groups:
- **People whose sexual partners are in or used to be in a HIV high risk category, including gay or bisexual men, intravenous drug users, prostitutes and their customers:** The incubation period, false negative test results, and predictable failure of resolutions to change behaviors combine to keep you at risk.

- **People who used to be in a high risk category and/ or have reason to believe they have been exposed to HIV:** Even though you may be successful in not returning to high risk behavior, the incubation period can cause you and your partner to be at risk. You both need to discuss all the facts and make ongoing decisions about your sexual sharing.
- **People who are in a committed sexual relationship with a partner who received a positive blood test for HIV antibodies or who has AIDS:** This can be a most difficult situation for both parties. You may err in consideration of your partner and may benefit from the objectivity of a counselor and/or support group.

GONORRHEA

Gonorrhea, commonly called the "clap", is a sexually transmitted disease caused by bacteria. According to the CDC, it is the second most common reported sexually transmitted disease in the United States (CDC, 2000). Women, 15 to 19 years old, and men, 20 to 24 years old, had the highest reported rate of gonorrhea.

When treated early, there are no long-term consequences of gonorrhea. Serious complications can result, however, when left untreated.

How it is Transmitted

Gonorrhea is spread by way of infected body fluids (semen, vaginal discharge, blood and ulcerations). It is almost always transmitted through sexual contact. Gonorrhea can occur in the reproductive organs, urethra, rectum and throat. It is also possible for pregnant women to pass the bacteria to their infant during birth.

Symptoms

Symptoms are not always present; fifty percent of persons with gonorrhea show no symptoms. Men are more likely than women to show signs of infection. If present, symptoms appear within 2 to 14 days.

Possible signs of Gonorrhea in Men:
- Painful urination
- Creamy or green, pus-like penile discharge
- Testicular pain

Possible signs of Gonorrhea in Women:
- Creamy or green, pus-like vaginal discharge
- Painful urination
- Bleeding between periods
- Excessive bleeding during menstrual period
- Painful intercourse
- Lower abdominal pain

Possible signs of Rectal infection:
- Itching
- Creamy, pus-like discharge
- Rectal bleeding
- Pain
- Constipation

Possible signs of Throat infection:
- Sore throat
- Swollen lymph glands
- Discharge

CHLAMYDIA

Chlamydia is a common and curable infection caused by bacteria. The bacteria target the cells of the reproductive organs, urethra, rectum, the lining of the eyelid and less commonly, the throat and rectum.

In the United States, chlamydia is the most commonly reported bacterial transmitted disease, particularly among sexually active adolescents and young adults. One in ten adolescent females test positive for Chlamydia. The number of cases among teenage girls, ages 14-19, continues to rise yearly (CDC, 2000).

How it is Transmitted

Chlamydia is passed primarily during anal or vaginal sex. It is less likely to be transmitted through oral sex. It can be passed when the mucous membrane, the soft skin covering all the openings of the body, comes into contact with the mucous membrane secretions or semen of an infected person.

During oral sex, it is possible but unlikely for chlamydia to be transmitted because the bacteria that cause chlamydia prefer to target the genital area rather than the throat.

Chlamydia can be passed even if the penis or tongue does not go all the way into the vagina or anus. If the vagina, cervix, anus, penis or mouth come in contact with infected secretions or fluids; then transmission is possible. Even a woman who has not had anal sex can get chlamydia in the anus or rectum if bacteria are spread from the vaginal area, such as when wiping with toilet paper. Eye infections in adults may result when discharge caries the disease into the eye during sex or hand-to-eye contact.

Chlamydia is not passed through things like shaking hands or toilet seats. Even if a person with chlamydia is treated and cured, they can be reinfected if they are exposed to chlamydia again. It can also be passed from mother to newborn as the baby passes through the infected birth canal. This can result in eye infections, pneumonia or other complications.

In children, chlamydia may be a possible sign of sexual abuse.

Symptoms

Approximately, seventy-five percent of women and fifty percent of men do not experience symptoms. If a person does have symptoms, they usually develop within one to three weeks after exposure to chlamydia. The period of infectivity is difficult to determine since so many people are asymptomatic. A person must be considered infectious (able to pass the bacteria along to others) from the time they become infected until treatment is completed. The symptoms of chlamydia are similar to the symptoms of gonorrhea and the two infections are often confused.

Both men and women can experience proctitis (inflamed rectum), urethritis (inflamed urethra) and conjunctivitis (inflamed eyelid). Most infections of the mouth and throat are asymptomatic. If present, symptoms are soreness and redness in the throat or mouth. The most common complications in newborns include conjunctivitis and pneumonia.

Most women are asymptomatic, but if symptoms are present they may be minor. Symptoms may include vaginal discharge and/or a burning sensation during urination.

If the infection spreads to the fallopian tubes, women

may experience: lower abdominal and lower back pain, pain during intercourse, bleeding between menstrual periods, nausea or fever.

Men may be asymptomatic or symptoms may be minor. When symptomatic, men may experience one or more of the following: Pus (thick yellow-white fluid) or watery or milky discharge from the penis, pain or burning during urination and/or pain or swelling of the testicles.

Because the symptoms of chlamydia are similar to the symptoms of gonorrhea, and because a person can be infected with both, the Centers for Disease Control and Prevention (CDC) recommends that people with chlamydia are treated for both diseases. Partners should be examined and treated as well (ASHA, 2001).

TRICHOMONIASIS (TRICH)

Trich is caused by a parasitic protozoa called Trichomonas. This parasite can survive for several hours on damp items such as towel and toilet seats. Trich itself is not known to lead to serious complications. However, when left untreated, trich can increase the risk of acquiring or transmitting AIDS (ASHA, 2001).

How it is Transmitted

Trich is passed from one person to another during vaginal sex.

Symptoms

Many men and women, who are infected, have no symptoms. Trich infects both men and women, but causes little or no symptoms in men.

Symptoms in women include:
- Unusual and increased vaginal discharge (bubbly, pale green, or gray) with an unpleasant odor
- Itching, burning, or redness of the vulva and vagina
- Pain during sex

GENITAL HERPES

Herpes is caused by the herpes simplex viruses type 1 (HSV -1) and type 2 (HSV-2).

HSV-1 and HSV-2 can be found and released from the sores that the viruses cause, but they also are released between episodes from skin that does not appear to be broken or to have a sore. A person almost always gets HSV-2 infection during sexual contact with someone who has a genital HSV-2 infection. HSV-1 causes infections of the mouth and lips, so-called "fever blisters." A person can get HSV-1 by coming into contact with the saliva of an infected person. HSV-1 infection of the genitals almost always is caused by oral-genital sexual contact with a person who has the oral HSV-1 infection.

Results of a recent, nationally representative study show that genital herpes infection is common in the United States. Nationwide, 45 million people ages 12 and older, or one out of five of the total adolescent and adult population, are infected with HSV-2.

HSV-2 infection is more common in women (approximately one out of four women) than in men (almost one out of five). This may be due to male-to-female transmission being more efficient than female-to-male transmission. HSV-2 infection also is more common in blacks (45.9%) than in whites (17.6%). Race and ethnicity in the United States correlate with other, more fundamental determinants of health such as poverty, access to good quality health care, behavior for seeking health care, illicit drug use, and living in communities with a high prevalence of STD's.

Since the late 1970's, the number of Americans with genital herpes infection has increased 30%. The largest increase is currently occurring in young white teens. HSV-2 infection is now five times more common in 12 to 19 year old whites, and it is twice as common in young adults ages 20 to 29 than it was 20 years ago.

HSV-2 can cause potentially fatal infections in infants if the mother is shedding virus at the time of delivery. It is important that women avoid contracting herpes during pregnancy because a first episode during pregnancy causes a greater risk of transmission to the newborn. If a woman has active genital herpes at delivery, a cesarean delivery is usually performed. Fortunately, infection of an infant from women with HSV-2 infection is rare.

In the United States, HSV-2 may play a major role in the heterosexual spread of HIV, the virus that causes AIDS. Herpes can make people more susceptible to HIV infection, and it can make HIV-infected individuals more infectious.

How it is transmitted

Herpes can be passed from one person to another when ulcerations contact mucosal surfaces (e.g., the male urethra, the vagina or cervix, the mouth, the anus, open wounds, etc.) and/or the skin.

Symptoms

Most individuals have no or only minimal signs or symptoms from HSV-1 or HSV-2 infection. When signs do occur, they typically appear as one or more blisters on or around the genitals or rectum. The blisters break, leaving tender ulcers (sores) that may take two to four weeks to heal the first time they occur. Other signs and symptoms during the primary episode may include a second crop of sores, or flu-like symptoms, including fever and swollen glands. Typically, another outbreak can appear weeks or months after the first, but it almost always is less severe and shorter than the first episode.

Although the infection can stay in the body indefinitely, the number of outbreaks tends to go down over a period of years. However, HSV-2 can cause recurrent painful genital sores in many adults, and HSV-2 infection can be severe in people with suppressed immune systems. Regardless of severity of symptoms, genital herpes frequently causes psychological distress in people who know they are infected.

SYPHILIS

Syphilis is a genital ulcerative disease cause by a bacteria. Syphilis can facilitate the transmission of HIV.

". . . it is now known that the genital sores caused by syphilis in adults also make it easier to transmit and acquire HIV infection sexually. There is a 2 to 5 fold increased risk of acquiring HIV infection when syphilis is present" (CDC, 2001). If left untreated, Syphilis can damage heart, brain, eyes, nervous system, bones and joints, resulting in blindness, heart disease and/or death.

The rate of syphilis increased slightly in 2001 and even more in 2002. The incidence of syphilis was highest among women aged 20-24 years and among men aged 35-39 (CDC, 2002).

How it is transmitted

Like herpes, syphilis can be passed from one person

to another when ulcerations, or the bacteria causing the ulcerations, contact mucosal surfaces (e.g., the male urethra, the vagina or cervix, the mouth, the anus, open wounds, etc.) and/or the skin. Transmission of the organism usually occurs during vaginal, anal, or oral sex. Pregnant women with the disease can pass it to the babies they are carrying.

T. pallidum, the baterium that causes syphilis, requires warm, moist environment, such as the genitals or the mucous membranes inside the mouth or anus, to survive. Syphilis cannot be spread by toilet seats, door knobs, swimming pools, hot tubs, bath tubs, shared clothing, or eating utensils.

Symptoms

The first symptoms of syphilis, or primary syphilis, appear 1-12 weeks after contact with infected partner. It is a small, red, pea-sized bump that soon develops into a round, painless sore called a chancre and appears on the site where the bacteria initially entered the body. It may go unnoticed and without treatment will disappear but the bacterium remains in the body and the person is highly contagious.

Left untreated it develops into secondary syphilis about 6 weeks after the chancre has disappeared. At this stage, the principal symptom is a skin rash that neither itches nor hurts. This rash may appear in the palms of the hands, the soles of the feet, or any other area on the body. Again, the person is still highly contagious.

Left untreated the symptoms disappear in two to six weeks, this is the latency period. The person remains contagious for approximately one year to sex partners; however, a pregnant woman can still infect her fetus.

Left untreated, tertiary syphilis develops which can be fatal.

HUMAN PAPILLOMAVIRUS (HPV)

Genital HPV infection is caused by human papillomavirus (HPV). Human papillomavirus, or HPV, is the name of a group of viruses that includes more than 100 different strains or types. Over 30 of these are sexually transmitted, and they can infect the genital area, like the skin of the penis, vulva, labia, or anus, or the tissues covering the vagina and cervix.

Approximately twenty million people are currently infected with HPV. Fifty to 75% of sexually active men and women acquire genital HPV infection at some point in their lives. About 5.5 million Americans get a new genital HPV infection each year (NIAID, 2001).

In the United States, HPV is considered to be one of the most prevalent sexually transmitted disease (STD). Some studies estimate that the majority of the sexually active population is exposed to at least one or more types of HPV - although most do not develop symptoms. Because HPV is so common and prevalent, a person does not need have to have a lot of sexual partners to come into contact with this virus (ASHA, 2001).

How it is transmitted

The types of HPV that infect the genital area are spread primarily through sexual contact. Most HPV infections have no signs or symptoms; therefore, most infected persons are completely unaware they are infected, yet they can transmit the virus to a sex partner. Rarely, pregnant women can pass HPV to their baby during vaginal delivery. A newborn that is exposed to HPV during delivery can develop warts in the larynx (voice box).

Symptoms

Most people who have a genital HPV infection do not know they are infected. The virus lives in the skin or mucus membranes and there are usually no symptoms. One study sponsored by the National Institute of Allergy and Infectious Diseases (NIAID) reported that almost half of the women infected with HPV had no obvious symptoms.

Some of these viruses are considered "high-risk" types and may cause abnormal Pap smears and cancer of the cervix, anus, and penis. Others are "low-risk," and they may cause mild Pap smear abnormalities and genital warts.

Genital warts usually appear as soft, moist, pink or red swellings. They can be raised or flat, single or multiple, small or large. Some cluster together forming a cauliflower-like shape. They can appear on the vulva, in or around the vagina or anus, on the cervix, and on the penis, scrotum, groin, or thigh. Warts can appear within several weeks after sexual contact with an infected person, or they can take months to appear.

Genital warts are diagnosed by inspection. Visible genital warts can be removed, but no treatment is better than another, and no single treatment is ideal for all cases.

Genital warts are very contagious and are spread during oral, genital, or anal sex with an infected partner. About two-thirds of people who have sexual contact with a partner with genital warts will develop warts, usually within three months of contact.

Most women are diagnosed with HPV on the basis of abnormal Pap smears. Pap smears are the primary screening tool for cervical cancer or pre-cancerous conditions, many of which are cell changes related to HPV. Current HPV tests are fairly sophisticated and expensive and are commercially available for women with an abnormal Pap smear. They cannot identify which HPV infections will lead to cervical cancer or pre-cancerous conditions. Research is underway to determine the role of HPV tests for cervical cancer screening.

There is no "cure" for HPV, although most infections usually go away on their own. Cancer-related types are more likely to persist.

CHAPTER THREE: RISK

Trust in the frailty of humanity.
Clark Taylor, Ph.D., Ed.D, M.P.H.

You can contract any STD by taking part in unsafe sex practices with someone who is infected. It does not matter if these are with men or women; gay, straight or bisexual; old, young or pregnant; your partner, spouse or lover.

The burden of responsibility for your sexual health lies within yourself. You must NEVER depend on anyone to be responsible for your health. It is important to always protect yourself and not allow others to persuade you to have unprotected sex. If your partner(s) does not want to practice safe sex, you still must protect yourself. If your partner(s) does not want you to protect yourself then maybe you need to find a partner(s) that will be more supportive about your health and well-being.

Trust in the frailty of humanity. You cannot rely on people to tell you the absolute truth when it comes to sex. People's sexuality is one of the most private aspects of their lives. Most people are reluctant, if not unwilling, to reveal their innermost sexual secrets. They may be embarrassed, ashamed, or feel that full disclosure might hurt their partner(s), restrict their freedom, and/or jeopardize their chances of a sexual encounter. To put it simply, sometimes they don't tell you critical information and sometimes they just lie!

Many people have been in situations, either directly or indirectly, that may put them at risk for STD's.

Some of these situations may include:

- Men who have sex with prostitutes even through they are in a committed relationship or married.
- Married men and women who have casual sex or ongoing sexual affairs with partner(s) outside of their primary relationship. These outside partners may or may not be having sex with others who may be engaged in risky behavior.
- Heterosexual women and men who have occasional or periodic sexual encounters with homosexual or bisexual men.
- A new sexual partner(s) who may be, or may have been, a needle sharing intravenous drug user.
- People who may have received a blood transfusion before the blood supply was tested and screened for contaminated blood.

Again, it is up to you to protect yourself! Remember, self-protection is part of self-love. If you are in a committed relationship or married, the trust bond implies but **does not guarantee full disclosure**. Many people associate arousal and passion with actions that are taboo (forbidden). You may have one-night stands and affairs for excitement because you are trained since childhood that this is what is exciting. The cookie jar effect!

Many people struggle with this issue. Casual sex, adolescent or young adult sexual activity and new sexual partners **do not lend themselves to full disclosure**.

The study, Sex, Lies and HIV, conducted on 665 southern California university students in 1990 and in the follow up studies at the University of Cincinnati in 1998 and 1999, show that sexual partners do not disclose, or would not disclose, to one another the truth about their past and current sexual relationships. Over 70% of men and women would not tell their partner if they were having sex with other partners. Also over 20% of the respondents would lie to their partner if they were HIV positive.

Few people actually know if they have been exposed to infections. Those who know they have been exposed are aware that if they share this information with someone they want to have sex with, they may be turned down.

Therefore, you are still at risk and need to practice safe sex even when:
- you know our sex partner
- you are monogamous
- you or your partner(s) have a negative antibody test for HIV
- you reduce the number of your sex partners.

Again, the message here is not about being distrustful and/or skeptical but to understand that people are human and humans make mistakes. **Most people are not out to harm others, but sometimes they do. The message is to be responsible for yourself and not to expect or depend on anyone else to be responsible for you, your health or your life.**

Basics for Risk Reduction

Approach safe sex from a place of empowerment. If you choose to have sex, you can do so without fear of pregnancy, disease and death if you follow a few basic and simple guidelines.

These guidelines are:
- Do not exchange bodily fluids
- Always use protection for vaginal, anal or oral sex
- Develop a low-stress lifestyle including physiological stress (drugs, alcohol, malnutrition, insomnia, overwork, pain) and psychological and emotional stress (worry, fear, anger, anxiety, doubt, depression,)
- Ask yourself these questions before having unprotected sexual activities with someone:
  - Would you engage in any of these activities with this person, without protection, if you knew they had one or more STD's including HIV/AIDS?
  - How can you know that they are free of infection?
  - Would you bet your "life" on it?

Developing Levels of Risk Reduction

A sexual encounter includes many distinct activities (e.g. touching, kissing, genital contact). Each of these activities has different possible risks attached to them and calls for different risk reduction strategies. Risk reduction strategies can be thought of as layers of protection against contact with STD's. It is important to have different strategies available for the same activity and it may be wise to use more than one layer of protection at the same time. The more types of risk reduction you incorporate into sex, the safer you will be.

If you do not come into contact with your partner's body fluids (example in mutual masturbation or using a condom), you will not come in contact with HIV and other discharge STD's and you won't have to worry about unwanted pregnancies.

You endanger your life everyday by getting into a car and driving somewhere. The chances of being killed in a car accident are much greater than dying from AIDS. Yet, you are not so terrified of driving that you refuse to leave the relative safely of your home. Instead you go through a variety of risk reduction strategies to reduce the chance of being involved in an accident. These include wearing seat belts, appropriately servicing the car, and, not speeding, not driving under the influence of alcohol or drugs, and driving defensively. This form of defensive driving is analogous to safer sex. The big difference is that with driving, even if you do everything right, some driver could run into you, causing pain and sometimes death. Not so with safe sex, if you take complete responsibility for being safe, you are in control.

The level of risk reduction that you choose is an individual decision based on your lifestyle, priority and scientific information. The inherent risk in every sexual encounter can be reduced in some way. It is your choice!

One of the highest risk behaviors for contracting HIV is anal intercourse. If you do not particularly like anal intercourse, it may be easiest for you to give up the behavior completely. If you have found that anal intercourse is particularly fun and pleasurable, you may choose to tolerate a higher risk by having anal sex in a safer way rather than just giving it up or doing it unsafely.

For example, you can engage in anal sex with the inserter wearing a condom. It might be even safer if the inserter wears two condoms. If the inserter pulls out just before ejaculation (wearing one or two condoms), it adds another layer of protection. The idea is to reduce the chance that, as much as possible in any given situation, you will not become infected.

If you are going to have responsible, safe and pleasurable sex, then it is to your advantage to expose yourself to as little risk as possible. For example, if you run out of condoms, gloves and dams, you could choose to play in other pleasurable, erotic and mutually satisfying ways that do not involve risk.

Safe Sex Guidelines

It is common to divide risk reduction guidelines into three categories.

These categories are:
- **Completely safe or no risk activities** present the least likelihood of STD transmission.
- **Probably safe or possibly risky activities** contain elements of possible risk or are activities about which there is insufficient knowledge and information.
- **Unsafe activities** that have been clearly linked to STD transmission.

The bottom line of all guidelines is that unprotected anal and vaginal intercourse and unprotected oral sex are proven to be high-risk behavior if the other person has STD's. And, that most of the time you do not know for certain if your partner is infected or has been exposed to infection. Therefore, these behaviors, without protection with anyone, are considered risky.

Safe or No Risk Activities

No exchange of body fluids / no contact with genital ulcerations diseases.

No risk activities include:
- Hugging
- Social (dry) kissing
- Bathing together
- Body massage
- Tasting own body fluid
- Body licking (non-genital on healthy clean skin)
- Masturbation (mutual or solitary)
- Personal sex toys
- S&M games (without bruising or bleeding)

Probably Safe, Possibly Risky Activities
Protected exchange of body fluids / protection from genital ulceration diseases.

Probably safe, possibly risky activities include:
- French kissing when partner has no mouth sores.
- Fellatio (oral-penile sex) without ejaculation with a condom
- Fellatio with ejaculation wearing a condom
- Cunnilingus (oral-vaginal sex) with a latex barrier
- Penile-vaginal intercourse with condom (safer with spermicide, safer yet when combined with a cervical barrier – diaphragm)
- Manual-anal sex (fingering or fisting the anus) with a latex glove
- Manual-vaginal sex with a latex glove
- Anal intercourse with condom (safer to withdraw before ejaculation)
- Analingus (anal-oral sex) with barrier protection
- Contact with urine (golden showers or water sports on unbroken skin)

Unsafe Activities
Exchange of body fluids / skin contact with genital ulceration diseases.

Unsafe activities include:
- Vaginal intercourse without a condom (even if the partner(s) pulls out)
- Anal intercourse without a condom (even if the partner(s) pulls out)
- Unprotected Fellatio (oral-penile sex)
- Unprotected Cunnilingus (oral-vaginal sex)
- Unprotected Analingus (anal-oral sex)
- Unprotected manual-anal sex (fingering or fisting the anus without a latex glove)
- Unprotected manual-vaginal sex (fingering or fisting the vagina without a latex glove)
- Contact with urine on broken skin
- Sharing menstrual blood
- Sharing needles or blood while piercing or shooting drugs

Risk increases with the number of partners in unprotected activities!

Risk also increases when people are drunk or high on drugs because they tend to act without thinking of the consequences! Probably the number one reason why people don't have safe sex, even though they want to, is due to the use of alcohol and other drugs. This book is not part of the anti-drug war. The fact is many people use drugs (and alcohol is a drug) and make poor decisions while under the influence.

Special Risk Factors

Safe sex guidelines are a general guide but the risk factors change depending on the situation. You must consider the particulars of every sexual encounter in order to use the guidelines correctly.

Your risk increases if you, or your partner(s), have:
- Cuts or broken skin
- A raw throat, sores in your mouths or bleeding gums
- Oral lesions (herpes I and II, syphilis and CMV ulcers)
- Genitals that are dry or irritated
- Untrimmed fingernails can make any digital intercourse riskier.
- Unplanned opportunistic sex
- A compromised immune system due to any infection (even minor ones - colds, flu)

CHAPTER FOUR: PROTECTION

*S*afe sex is the most important deterrent you have against any STD. The key guideline remains: **don't share blood (this includes menstrual blood), semen, rectal or vaginal fluids, and use barrier protection every time there is anal, vaginal or oral sex.**

Saying "no" to sex is not the only answer, in fact, for most people it is not even an option. Saying a firm and powerful "NO!" to any potential partner who does not want to practice safe sex is a must in preventing STD's.

Sex should be about pleasure and fun - not fear. All partners should come away from the experience feeling sexually satisfied as well as disease free. Practicing safe sex will help dissolve fear and heighten satisfaction and pleasure.

There are many options for safety. The more strategies or layers of risk reduction you use, the greater your chances are that you will insure protection.

It is important to discuss your desire to use protection before you start having sex. Make it an extension of your usual sex play so that things go smoothly. Let yourself be creative! Think up new ways to incorporate safety into your sex life can be fun and very sexy. Talking about protection is extremely helpful and becomes easy with practice. Be honest about your feelings. If you are nervous, embarrassed and inexperienced, you need to say so! It gives you room to experiment and gives an unspoken permission for your partner(s) to be honest too. It also gives your partner a chance to explore, share tales of latex delights or nightmares, and/or deal with negative feelings, doubts an fears before you are in the middle of having sex.

Some people find that being very direct is the best way to approach safe sex. You might say, "I use protection, how about you?" Some people love this kind of talk and some hate it. Make your approach fit your style and the occasion.

Again, if a partner refuses to use, or allow you to use, protection, don't fight it – do things that are low risk or, better yet, find another partner because any partner that does not respect your rights and desire for protection does not deserve to be intimate with you!

Spermicides and Microbicides

In 1992, Dr. Ted McIlvenna wrote a memo pointing out that using condoms alone was like playing Russian roulette because one out of six condoms used are defective either though product failure or human error. Also, in that same memo, Dr. McIlvenna took a look at how the policy of the government, at that time, was an "anti-sexual one." He goes on to say, "Denial and abstinence are considered the ideal, even though the facts of sexual behavior continue to prove over and over again that the official government position is at best ill-informed and at worse ridiculous."

Now, in 2003, the situation is even worse with President Bush's abstinence-only-until-marriage campaign. Dr. McIlvenna's message about your greatest hope being "education that is realistic and sex-positive" and that "eroticizing safer sex is your best line of protection" is timeless.

In June 2000, the National Institute of Health (NIH), in collaboration with the Centers for Disease Control and Prevention (CDC), the Food and Drug Administration (FDA), and the United States Agency for International Development (USAID), convened a workshop to evaluate the published evidence establishing the effectiveness of latex male condoms in reducing the risks of STD's, including HIV.

The result of the studies showed that "correct and consistent use of the male latex condom can *reduce the risk* (emphasis added) of STD transmission" (CDC, 2002).

You do not want to "reduce the risk" of transmission, you want to *prevent it*! Therefore, a new strategy of protection is recommended. In 1992, The Institute of Advanced Study of Human Sexuality proposed a campaign of **"When you do it – Lube it!"** It is time to reinstate this message!

Sharing the Front Line of Defense

At the beginning of the AIDS epidemic, the IASHS made a plea to government and private industry to unite in developing HIV topical microbicides, stating that the creation of a truly effective product (or combination of products) would render an invaluable service to humanity. Now the Institute feels more strongly than ever about developing topical microbicides as a necessary line of defense.

Chemoprophylaxis (Universal Prophylaxis)

Chemoprophylaxis is a drug treatment designed to prevent future occurrences of disease. Treatment for the entire population as a whole is called chemoprophylactic. This is what is needed in the battle against STD's.

The Need for Topical Microbicides

The various substances that kill STD's or inhibit disease transmission during sex are called "topical microbicides." Unfortunately, this is still one of the most neglected areas of prevention research. The development of antibiotics that cured some STD's stunted the development of topical microbicides. No one seemed to care about prevention when there was a drug to "cure." However, when herpes and HIV became epidemics with no "cure" in sight, prevention, once again, became a burning issue.

Research now is becoming more sexologically sophisticated. Researchers are starting to pay attention to such factors as taste, smell and feel of products used for sex. Unfortunately, however, researchers still usually concentrate only on one sexual option - peno-vaginal intercourse. Since sexually transmitted diseases are commonly transmitted through anal sex, oral sex and injured skin as well as coitus, vaginal products are not generally designed to provide the over-all protection people need to prevent HIV/STD transmission.

To be effective, a topical microbicide must coat all mucosal surfaces exposed to infection. This means inserting a given amount of product inside the body. The amount depends upon the spreading and adhesive qualities of the product, concentration of microbicides and many other factors.

Unfortunately, there is a wide range of product sophistication and product integrity with little guidance or support from the government or mainstream AIDS/ STD researchers to improve lubricant quality. Indeed, as governmental agencies have become aware of the tremendous potential of sexual lubricants, the tendency has been to retard product development rather than encourage and support the industry. The company that the Institute feels deserves recognition for their continuing research and development of sensuous, effective sexual lubricants is Taylor-Wright Pharmacals.

Researchers and health educators are looking into different agents capable of killing HIV and other STD's on contact. Thus it might be that a foam, cream or gel with inert and antiseptic ingredients already approved and sold over the counter might be more effective against AIDS than any of the detergent products presently available.

Microbicides are especially needed to protect women. And, attention to the prevention and treatment of STD's among women is lacking even though the CDC in its 2001 STD Surveillance Report on STD's in Women and Children stated a significant increase in cases of all STD's among women (CDC, 2001).

> In spite of the tremendous public attention that HIV/AIDS has received and the commitment of both public and private funds to AIDS research, little attention has been given to the need for a woman-initiated form of STD prevention. Research efforts in women's health have been severely under-funded and tend to ignore social realities that women face.
>
> (RHTP, 2001-02).

There are also questions about the most effective way to use a microbicide rectally. For example, to be effective, a microbicide should remain in the vagina for 4 or 5 hours after intercourse and women are advised not to douche. However, after anal intercourse, it is common to have a bowel movement. Must the microbicide be reapplied in such cases? And how long must the microbicide remain in the' bowel to be maximally effective? It may be that for anal use, because of the delicate membranes and the limited natural secretions, a different combination of inert ingredients will be required.

Obviously, the amount of a microbicide required to kill HIV depends in part upon the nature of the overall product. Those products that spread well and also create a physical barrier to transmission will not need as much detergent.

Nonoxynol-9

If nonoxynol-9 were a completely effective form of prevention, the situation would not be so urgent. However the commercial grade of nonoxynol-9 used in most products contains impurities that are sometimes irritating and can damage cell membranes. As well, some researchers have proven that high concentrations of nonoxynol-9 removes the mucosa from the vagina and rectum and thus leaves it more vulnerable to any virus.

N-9 had been widely used for more than 30 years in over-the-counter gels, foams, creams and films designed to kill sperm and it is still being used as a contraceptive for women.

Researchers have shown that N-9 can kill HIV and other STD microbes in laboratory experiments. Previous studies in small numbers of women suggested that N-9 had some benefit as a topical microbicide, a virus and bacteria killing product that women can apply into her vagina before having sex. However, researchers also have been concerned that frequent use or high doses of N-9 could disrupt the cells that line the genital tract, thereby increasing the chances of HIV infection.

A NIAID sponsored clinical trial was conducted by Family Health International (FHI) in Cameroon to evaluate the efficacy of a vaginal film containing N-9 in blocking HIV among 1,300 female sex workers in two cities in Cameroon from 1996 –2000.

Almost two years into the study a preliminary analysis was released and showed the overall rate of HIV transmission to be 6.7 percent, half the transmission rate that was previously estimated in this population. This rate reduction was the same in both the N-9 film users and the placebo group.

"We are encouraged by the apparent effectiveness of the overall intervention program that included counseling, STD treatment and encouragement of condom use," says Rodney Hoff, Ph.D., chief of the efficacy trials branch in NIAID's AIDS Vaccine Research and Prevention Program. "We nevertheless had hoped that the N-9 film might increase a woman's available options for HIV and STD protection." However, by the end of the study the infection rate was 50% higher in the N-9 group (NIAID, 2000).

Because of these results, and the results of other studies, The Food and Drug Administration (FDA) is proposing new labeling warning statements for all over-the-counter (OTC) vaginal contraceptive drug products containing N-9. These warning statements will advise consumers that vaginal contraceptives containing N-9 do not protect against infection from HIV, the virus that causes acquired immunodeficiency syndrome (AIDS), or against getting other STD's. The warnings will also advise consumers that frequent use of vaginal contraceptives containing N-9 can increase vaginal irritation. Increased vaginal irritation from use of N-9 may increase the possibility of transmission of the AIDS virus (HIV) and STD's from infected partners (Dotzel, 2002).

The women who used N-9 had a high incidence of vaginal lesions. Studies have consistently shown that liaisons are a breading area for infection (CDC, 2000).

Using a high percentage of N-9 on the delicate mucosa of the vagina can be compared to douching with TIDE! This form of irritation kills vaginal-wall cells, causing ulceration and thus giving the virus an entry-point.

On top of that if you add the factor of multiple intercourse because of the nature of their trade and you can logically see how the study failed to give anything but poor results.

ForPlay's Inter-Lube

A low percentage of N-9 has been used, for a better part of three years, with sex workers in Southern California at the AIM clinic. The testing was arranged, by the Institute of Advanced of Human Sexuality, as a research project in conjunction with the Trimensa Company, who provides the product to AIM at no cost. The product that was used, and continues to be used, is Inter-Lube from Trimensa's ForPlay line. Inter-Lube contains 0.1% N-9 as its active ingredient. The women use Inter-Lube every 24 hours, and sometimes more often, with no douching. AIM reports no irritation and no new cases of Chlamydia and Gonorrhea. AIM stopped using Inter-Lube for a period of several months, and during that time there was a high rate of new infections. Once the Inter-Lube program was restarted, AIM once again reported no new cases of Chlamydia and Gonorrhea. This low percentage (0.1% N-9) appears to kill STD's but has not yet been tested as a spermicide.

Erogel

Since 1978 the Institute for Advanced Study of Human Sexuality has been involved in a research project with members of the adult sex industry.

In the early 1980's, The Institute along with the Mariposa Foundation and Trimensa Corporation conducted testing on 3 female sex workers. These sex workers were infected with a treatable and curable strain of gonorrhea. One hundred men were recruited for a double blind cross over study using a 3% solution of N-9 with vaginal penetration. The results showed that N-9 was effective in the prevention of gonorrhea, however 21 of the men had minor reactions to N-9 and 3 of the men had noticeable reactions. During this time AIDS became know and the study was to continue to test for other contact kill factors however, for possible political reasons, the study ended abruptly.

In 1982, the Institute looked into a formula to keep the microbicide effects of N-9 but buffer the solution so there would be no irritation. The result was a formula consisting of nonoxynol-15, a detergent-based product, similar to that of nonoxynol-9, and a homeopathic buffering agent, Avena Sativa. The product was Erogel.

The Institute tested this product initially on 100 female sex workers. These workers were encouraged to use condoms along with the Erogel however, many sex workers do not use condoms. After 2 years into the study 71 of the workers were still actively working in the industry, still using Erogel and still disease free. Erogel was also used in 190 sex films and 8 swing clubs. The Department of Public Health was called in to do the testing, and everyone using the product was free of all STD's and irritation.

This is how it works: Erogel, because of its detergent base, forms and spreads over the mucosa of the vagina, giving overall protection. Plus, it is slippery and wet – a great personal lubricant.

The success of this product is overwhelming. Because HIV is it chronic and progressive, there cannot be a double blind study. However it has been tested for years with members of the adult sex industry and, in all cases, no one using Erogel has contracted any STD's, including HIV. Additionally, women had a history of severe reactions to nonoxynol-9 had no negative reactions.

Erogel has not been tested exclusively for anal intercourse; therefore you cannot recommend this, or any other product, for that use. This product currently has a soapy taste and is in the process of being tested for flavorings and still be effective with contact kill. Erogel has also being tested as a spermicide with great success.

Erogel is currently available for sale as a personal lubricant in most adult outlets and in many stores online. It cannot be sold as a mircobicide until all testing has been completed. Taylor-Wright Pharmacals is providing samples of this product through the Institute of Advanced Study of Human Sexuality's Research Department. You can try a free sample of this product, by including a note asking for a free sample of Erogel and a check for $5.00 for postage and handling, to IASHS, Research Department, 1523 Franklin Street, San Francisco, CA 94109.

Other Microbicides Being Tested

There are other products being tested as microbicides and spermicides. At the present time, there nearly 200 products being tested.

These products, that are in advanced stages of research, are:
- Carraguard
- PRO 2000/5 Gel
- BufferGel
- PMPA Gel

Carraguard

Carraguard is the proprietary name of a substance made from carrageenan, a carbohydrate gel derived from seaweeds that is widely used as a stabilizer in the food industry. Carrageenan contains large negatively charged molecules called sulphated polysaccharides. It is believed that their strong electric charges attract them either to the viruses (thus inactivating them) or to the cells of the vaginal wall (thus covering those cells like a coat of paint and preventing viruses from entering the body). Tests on animals suggest that the substance may offer similar protection against other STD's, including herpes, gonorrhoea and genital warts.

Carraguard has several things going for it. First, carrageenan is already known to America's Food and Drug Administration. The FDA has classified it as "generally recognized as safe", its highest safety rating. Second, Carraguard has shown no harmful effects in the early human trials.

Carraguard's third advantage, or disadvantage, is that it is not a spermicide. This offers greater choice to couples who want children (Economist, 2002).

Carraguard is due to come to market by 2006.

Pro2000/5 Gel

In 1998, Procept, Inc. presented findings at the 12th World AIDS Conference in Geneva showing that its vaginal microbicide, PRO 2000 Gel, may provide protection against a number of sexually transmitted diseases.

Procept scientists and colleagues described in vitro experiments showing that the antiviral compound PRO 2000 blocks infection by vaginal herpes simplex virus (HSV) types 1 and 2 and Chlamydia trachomatis. They also reported on the first in vivo evidence of PRO 2000 Gel's efficacy against an STD -- namely, findings that the gel provides complete protection against HSV-2 infection in mice.

HSV-2 infection is a significant public health problem, and genital herpes lesions may provide a portal of entry for human immunodeficiency virus (HIV) (Aegis, 1998).

BufferGel

RePprotect's flagship product as a vaginal microbicide is BufferGel™, which maintains the mild, protective acidity of the vagina. It is the first vaginal product designed to block the alkaline nature of semen. The vagina is naturally acidic (pH 4), which kills not only sperm, but also inactivates certain pathogens. Testing is being done to see if BufferGel™ will offer some protection against unwanted pregnancy and STD's, including HIV, by enhancing a natural protective function of the vagina.

Unlike vaginal spermicides now on the market, BufferGel™ is detergent-free. It is a non-irritating, lubricant made of a Carbopol gel (Carbopol 974P), which is a high molecular weight, cross-linked, polyacrylic acid. Over the past 40 years, Carbopol has an outstanding record for safety in over one hundred pharmaceuticals for mucosal contact. BufferGel™ is an aqueous gel that is osmotically balanced with physiological salts. It contains no oil and is compatible for use with condoms and latex diaphragms.

BufferGel™ has gone through extensive pre-clinical testing and has been found to inhibit pregnancy, HIV transmission, human papilloma virus (HPV), herpes simplex virus (HSV), and chlamydia infections, without damaging the reproductive epithelium or microflora.

Two clinical trials have been completed on BufferGel™

used vaginally by women of reproductive age who were HIV-negative, and either sexually-active and monogamous with low risk for HIV acquisition, or sexually abstinent.

One trial was conducted in the United States; the other was conducted at four separate international sites: Pune, India; Chiang-Mai, Thailand; Blantyre, Malawi; and Harare, Zimbabwe. The majority of the participants in the studies said they would use the product if it were commercially available. Phase II/III data on BufferGel's contraceptive activity are expected in 2004; data on the anti-HIV activity of BufferGel™ are expected in 2005 (ReProtect, 2002).

New Clinical Trials on BufferGel and Pro 2000/5 Gel

A study on the Effects of BufferGel and PRO 2000/5 Gel in Men is being sponsored by National Institute of Allergy and Infectious Diseases (NIAID) to find out if there are any bad effects when BufferGel or PRO 2000/5 Gel when applied to the penis of HIV-infected men. Studies have shown 2 investigational microbicides, BufferGel and PRO 2000/5 Gel, to be safe and acceptable for women and HIV-negative men. It is important to see if the side effects of these products are the same in men as those in women and to see if there is any difference in the side effects between circumcised and uncircumcised men (Clinical Trials, 2003).

PMPA Gel

A study on the Safety and Acceptability of the Anti-Microbe Vaginal Gel, PMPA Gel, is being sponsored by National Institute of Allergy and Infectious Diseases (NIAID). The purpose of this study is to evaluate the PMPA gel, which kills microbes, in HIV-infected and HIV-uninfected women. The majority of new HIV infections occur through heterosexual contact. A product that stops or slows the replication of HIV during sexual contact is needed. At present, no products are completely effective.

PMPA gel, also known as tenofovir, is an anti-microbe agent that may fight against sexual transmission of HIV and other sexually transmitted diseases (STD's). It is applied to the vagina and gives women the ability to control their disease-prevention activity. (HPTN, 2003)

Condoms

Condoms are extremely important weapons in the war against STD's. To make the best of condoms you must use them properly, use them all the time and learn to enjoy them.

Using Condoms Correctly

Practice makes perfect. The main reason condoms fail is incorrect use. New condoms seldom leak or break due to faulty manufacturing.

Instructions for condom use are simple but must be followed carefully:

1. **Use condoms every time** you have vaginal, oral and/ or anal intercourse. Condoms are a main part of the line of protection. If you have a partner who gives you an argument here are some bottom line suggestions from Condomania, to put the most unwilling partner in their place. (Condomania, 2001)
   - *"I'm not available without one."*
   - *"No balloon, no party."*
   - *"No gown, no ball."*

2. **Keep a convenient supply of condoms in a cool, dry place**.

3. **Do not test condoms** by inflating or stretching them.
4. **Open the package carefully.** Rough handling and long and/or jagged nails can damage condoms.
5. **Gently press any air out** of the receptacle tip at the closed end before putting on the condom.
6. **Adding a dab of lubricant in the tip** will solve the air problem and greatly increase sensation.
7. **Unroll the condom so that it covers the entire penis.**
8. **When a man is uncircumcised,** the foreskin should be pulled back before covering the head with the condom. This will increase sensation.
9. **An erect penis insures the best fit.**
10. **If the penis is soft, unroll the entire condom down to the base as it hardens.**
11. **Do not insert penis beyond the condom base** as this can cause the condom to come off.
12. **Push back the public hair at the base of the penis**, this will help keep it from getting tangled in the condom.
13. **Use plenty of water-soluble lubricant** on the outside of the condom and on the vagina or anus before entry. Areas that are too dry can pull condoms off and tear them as well.
14. **Do not use oil-based lubricants**, like baby oil, Crisco and Vaseline because they cause the latex to break down and the condom to break. Some topical medications and vaginal creams contain oil.
15. **Hold on to the base of the condom when necessary.** If the penis is getting soft or the partner to very tight, the condom may tend to slip.

16. **Certain sexual positions tend to cause slipping.** For example, when a women is sitting on top of a man, the lips of her vulva can lift off the condom. Holding the base of the condom will solve the problem.
17. **After ejaculation, hold the condom at the base to avoid spilling or losing condom inside the partner.**
18. **Withdraw gently.**
19. **Throw used condoms away!**
20. **NEVER go from one person to another without changing condoms.**
21. **NEVER go from one opening to another (example anus to vagina) on the same person without changing condoms.**

Pick the condom that is right for you

When looking for the "right" condom, it is important to experiment!!!! You can try out lots of different kinds using low risk activities such as masturbation. You need to purposefully break some so you know how much stress they can take and what it feels like when a condom is torn.

Fit

With condoms, *exact size isn't everything!* Latex hugs and stretches to fit many sizes. Condoms, which fit snugly, slightly constrict the superficial veins of the penis making erections harder and orgasms more intense. Sex therapists often suggest this approach to men who are having trouble maintaining an erection during sex. Condoms with more room at the top allow the end of the condom to move and thus create more sensation. Length is not critical so long as the condom goes all the way to the base of the penis and people are careful during intercourse not to penetrate beyond where the condom ends.

Some people have tremendous fear that condoms will come off during sex. Further, because of the variety in penis shapes and sizes a few men do have a serious problem finding a condom brand that will stay on well. Occasionally, the condom will be gripped by the vaginal or rectal muscles and the penis will move in and out of the condom. This can feel good but runs the risk of losing the condom. When the condom begins to slip, you need to use your hands to "get a grip."

Thickness

Some condoms are thicker than others but modern production techniques have led to condoms of reduced thickness without sacrificing essential strength required by federal standards.

Age of condoms

More important than thickness for strength is the *age* of the condom and the way it is treated before and during use. Condoms have a shelf life of 5 years under optimal conditions but begin to deteriorate slowly after 2 1/2 years. Buy from a distributor who has a good turnover. Condoms also age quickly from heat, strong light and rough treatment. Don't leave them in the sun or keep them in car glove compartments. And don't keep them in billfolds for long periods. Packages made of foil or opaque plastic protect condoms much better that ones that have "see-through" covers.

Shapes

Condoms with receptacle tips to catch the ejaculate are recommended over rounded ends, but both are fine.

Condoms which have a mushroom top provide more

sensation to the head of the penis by allowing it freedom of movement and more comfortable for larger glans.

Ribbed condoms have little nubbies on the outside that can provide added sensation to the condom wearer's partner. Some like this and others find it irritating. You can try switching from ribbed to unribbed if your partner has had enough extra stimulation.

Colors, Tastes and Smells

People occasionally object at first to the taste or smell of latex, but after a few experiences with condoms and enjoyable sex most people find the taste and smell of latex an erotic turn on. Latex itself actually has very little taste. Additives make condom brands distinct. Also, you can consider flavored condoms as an option. Again, you can experiment and have fun.

You must be careful about condoms that are scented as the perfume can cause allergies. There is considerable variety in the taste, smell and flavor of condom lubricants so you can pick what you like the best. Though most colored condoms are fine, a few have unstable dyes and run. Pastel colors are better than the real bright ones.

Lubricated condoms

Lubricated condoms do not break as easily as un-lubricated ones. They also give a moist natural sexual feeling to the skin that the dry ones do not. This creates greater sensation for the wearer.

Condoms are lubricated with gels or silicone-based lubricants. Gels coat prophylactics unevenly inside the package, while silicone products lubricate all parts of the condom equally. The silicone coating is less gooey when the package is opened and the thorough wetness means they are less likely to break from grabbing on dry spots during use.

Some condoms are lubricated with nonoxynol-9 (see details on nonoxynol-9 under *Spermicides/Microbicides*). These are advertised as having a spermicidal lubricant.

Important considerations in choosing to use lubricated condoms are:

- They may or may not provide a minimum of local protection against STD's in case the condom breaks, leaks or spills.
- Nonoxynol-9 lubricated condoms have only been tested for vaginal intercourse.
- Some people find nonoxynol-9 mildly irritating. Nonoxynol-9 products should be tried out first, using low risk activities before taking a chance on becoming chapped and creating a possible route for infection. Most problems with irritation can usually be solved by simply changing brands. For that matter, the amount of nonoxynol-9 lubricant on these condoms is so minimal that irritation is generally non-existent.

Learn To Enjoy Condoms

Take your time and learn to use condoms properly.

You can learn to enjoy condoms by:

- Experimenting all you want. If you're clumsy, you don't have to sweat it. If you make a mess, you can open another one and start over again. If the going is easy, that's fine too.
- Keeping several types and sizes around so that you and/or your partner(s) will have a choice.

- Putting your favorite fantasy partners into condom scenes while you masturbate. Thinking up ways you might get these partners to use condoms and what it would be like.
- Testing out condom strength. Stretching them your arms length or getting a friend to help put a condom on your head. Blowing them up like balloons.
- You can't make condoms feel the exact same way as naked skin. But you can explore the sensations of latex. Once you do this, condoms often become extremely enjoyable - more like sexual enhancers than devices for sexual hygiene.
- There are a thousand ways to make putting on condoms an exciting part of sex instead of an interruption; one example is learning to put a condom on with your mouth. Pressing the reservoir tip between the lips and using the mouth, in an "O" shape to push the condom down over the "penis" (cucumbers or dildos can be substituted for the real thing for practice). Using the tongue and the hand as a guide and being especially careful of teeth. Perfecting this erotic technique will make your partner forget that you are even putting the condom on.
- Trying a taste test to choose the best tasting condom on the market.
- Use flavored lubes to add to the taste of using condoms for oral sex.
- Using as many condoms during sex as you like. Men often make the mistake of thinking that once they've put a condom on they have to ejaculate or else. Take your time and play and remember to change condoms when you change openings.

- Condoms cut down on friction and make some guys last longer before ejaculating. This is a wonderful feature of latex for many men and women, but a problem for others. If you don't want to make sex last longer, you can use other low risk options until you're close to ejaculation and then put on a condom.
- If you want, you can see for yourself what happens to a condom when you use an oil-based lubricant. Blow up two condoms. On one, rub a water-based lubricant, on the other you can use something oil based, for example Vaseline or baby oil. What you'll find is the condom with the Vaseline or the baby oil will explode in under a minute, the condom with the water-based lube will still be kicking around the next day.
- Using additional water-soluble lubricant. The lubrication on condoms helps but usually is not enough. You can heighten enjoyment by pouring just a little bit of lubricant into the reservoir tip before putting a condom on. This helps keep air out of the tip and greatly increases sensation when the lubricant seeps around the glans. It takes a little practice to get the right amount down, but is well worth the effort!
- Even the best water-soluble lubricants dry out during use. But if you wet them again, they're as good as new. Although saliva will work, it is not particularly hygienic. One solution is to have a glass of water around or a squeeze bottle, sprayer or bowl.
- In addition to the above suggestions, you can ask other people who use condoms how they have learned to enjoy them the most. Sharing experiences with your friends and being creative and coming up with your own techniques, adds to the enjoyment.

Why Condoms Don't Work and What To Do About It!

The major reason condoms fail to prevent disease is that people only use them part of the time. Wear them every time! Researchers state that the most common reasons most people give for not wearing condoms are:

- You think your partner is not infected
- You don't think condoms really work
- You forget to carry them
- You are too embarrassed to bring the subject up, afraid a partner will be offended
- You are too drunk or high on drugs to remember, care, or even be able to use them.

You don't want this to happen to you! If you're going to have sex, you must be prepared, willing and able to use protection!

The second most important reason condoms don't prevent disease is they leak or break. Sometimes a condom is poorly manufactured. More often, they leak or break because they are old and/or have been exposed to strong sunlight, heat or extreme cold. But the most common reasons are rough treatment and oil-based lubricants. **Never use oil-based lubricants on latex.**

Condoms only cover the penis and therefore only protect the organ and what it touches. You must be careful that infected body fluids do not get into cuts, abrasions, ingrown hairs, pimples, bleeding gums or other broken skin may spread the disease. Also, you must be careful to protect yourself and your partner from contact with any lesions (herpes, syphilis, warts) that may not be covered by the condom. You must be sure to check out your body and your partner's body to avoid unnecessary risks.

If a condom breaks during intercourse, you need to stop, urinate, clean up well and use a new condom. If ejaculation has occurred, partners **should not douche** as this can create small tears and spread possible infection.

If a condom breaks after ejaculation and you know your partner is infected you can call your health center about Post-exposure prophylaxis (PEP)

Post-Exposure Prophylaxis (PEP)

Post-exposure prophylaxis (PEP) is the use of antiviral drugs as soon as possible after exposure to HIV, to prevent HIV infection. PEP can reduce the rate of infection in health care workers exposed to HIV by 79%.

The benefits of PEP for non-occupational exposure *have not been proven*. This use of PEP is controversial because some people fear it will encourage unsafe behaviors.

PEP is a four-week program of two or three antiviral medications, several times a day. The medications have serious side effects that can make it difficult to finish the program. PEP is not 100% effective; it cannot guarantee that exposure to HIV will not become a case of HIV infection. (AIDS, 2001)

Other Forms of Protection

- *Diaphragms.* A diaphragm is a cup shaped device that covers a woman's cervix. While the diaphragm by itself is not a complete barrier against infection, it is an important addition to the safe sex arsenal. The first step is to make sure that the diaphragm fits correctly. The diaphragm, which holds a microbicide/spermicide, blocks the cervix (the neck of the uterus that projects into the vagina). By blocking the cervix germs are unable to gain entry into the uterus, which is easily accessible to the blood supply. It is recommended that the diaphragm be used in conjunction with other forms of barrier protection.

- *Latex and plastic examination gloves* are superb for anal play, clitoral and vaginal stimulation, body massage and other delights. They come plain, powdered or lubricated and in many different sizes, colors, and tastes. Gloves can be bought individually at many pharmacies and can be obtained in quantity from almost all surgical supply stores without a prescription. They can also be purchased online and at local adult toy stores. Make sure to remove rings and keep fingernails trimmed and smooth and use plenty of water-based lubricant. Also, use a different finger for each orifice and don't share or reuse.

- *Rubber dams* are squares of latex used by dentists to create a barrier to blood, saliva and germs during dental procedures. They are usually scented and/or flavored and make an excellent addition to any safe sex kit. Latex dams prevent the exchange of bodily fluids during oral sex. To use them, rinse off talc because it can cause irritation. Hold the dam over the vulva or anus during oral sex and make sure to keep it in place. Do not share or reuse. Dams are available at many safe sex and adult sexually-oriented stores and most dental supply stores. Or you can try cutting an unrolling a condom down one side and opening it up. You can use this as a dam during oral sex, Also, plastic kitchen wraps, while not tested or approved for this purpose, makes a larger and more versatile dam.

- *Latex finger cots* or latex finger condoms. Finger condoms offer protection from exposure due to chapped skin and/or torn cuticles during fingering or fisting of the vagina or anus. Make sure to remove rings and keep the fingernails trimmed and smooth and use plenty of water-based lubricants. Also, be sure and use a different finger cot for each orifice and don't share or reuse.

Female Condoms

The Female Health Company owns the worldwide rights to the female condom. In the United States and Canada it used to be marketed under the name "Reality" and in the rest of the world under the name "Femidom." This product is currently being marketed in the US with the name "Female Condom."

While the FDA says that you can expect a 84% effectiveness rating for the female condom there is some controversy about this with some. The Female Health Company believes this condom is under rated because of an inherent bias towards male applied condoms. With "perfect" usage, efficacy may go up to as much as 95%, which fits nicely with the figures for "perfectly" applied male condoms, but this figure should not be relied upon. It should be noted that the condom is relatively new to the market and because it is a new technology the methodology for testing it may not be as complete as that for latex condoms.

As with any form of barrier protection, the "Female Condom" is most effective used in conjunction with other forms of protective barriers and is currently the only female applied condom choice a woman has to protect herself from STD's when she is sexually active.

Neither the CDC nor the FDA, to date, has studied the use of the female condom for male on male anal sex but it is being used that way in the gay community. (Staube, 2002).

Protectaid® Contraceptive Sponge

The Protectaid® contraceptive sponge is a barrier device made of polyurethane foam impregnated with F-5 Gel®. F-5 Gel® is a spermicide that contains three agents; Nonoxynol-9 (N-9), Benzalkonium Chloride (BKC), and Sodium Cholate (NACOL). These are used in low concentrations to try to minimize the risk of cervical and vaginal irritation and irritation to the penis. Studies with Protectaid® have shown an absence of significant colposcopic irritation after 6-12 hour use periods. The F-5 Gel® was also shown to exert its spermicidal activity in vitro even when diluted. The individually wrapped disposable sponge is ready to use and designed with die-cut slots for easy insertion and removal.

The sponge provides protection for a 12 hour period and a new sponge is not required if multiple acts of intercourse occur during this period. The sponge is to be left in for a minimum of 6 hours after intercourse. In clinical tests, the overall efficiency rate was 90 percent. Condomania says it is their most popular item. The sponge is a very convenient form of contraception. There is no prescription or fitting required and insertion does not interrupt foreplay. It cannot be felt by either partner and there is no leakage after ejaculation because the sponge absorbs semen.

Studies on Protectaid® confirm contraceptive efficacy and preliminary studies indicate that the Protectaid® sponge may also help prevent STD's, including HIV. Though still to be confirmed in clinical studies, it is already well established that at least two of the active ingredients -- Nonoxynol-9 (N-9) and Benzalkonium Chloride (BKC) -- have strong virucidal, fungicidal and bactericidal activities. In vitro studies conducted by Axcan Ltd. demonstrated that the F-5 Gel®

destroys a large number of pathenogenic microorganisms including HIV, Chlamydia and the bacteria responsible for gonorrhea.

It is recommended that the sponge be used in conjunction with condoms for additional STD protection.

Other Helpers

There are many other items that can easily create an effective barrier for STD's or actually kill HIV on contact.

Some of these should not be placed on or in a person's body, but have a use in overall AIDS prevention.

- *Diaper wipes* often contain nonoxynol-9, alcohol and benzylkonium chloride (a substance which also kills. HIV). These wipes are excellent for cleaning up during and after sex. They are great for helping take off condoms! Read the ingredients. Some have aloe vera in them to keep skin from drying out.
- *Ordinary soaps and detergents* are very effective at killing the virus and should be used for cleaning up before and after sex and for cleaning sex toys.
- *Hydrogen peroxide* can be purchased from pharmacies to be used as a gargle and for disinfecting sores or wounds. Though hydrogen peroxide comes from the bottle in a 3% solution, it kills the virus quickly even when diluted with water as low as 10 parts and can be used in many creative ways. For example it can be freshly diluted and used as an added layer of protection when rewetting water-soluble lubricants.
- *Diluted household bleach* (1 part bleach, 10 parts water) is excellent for cleaning many sex toys and cleaning up playrooms after sex.

- *Plastic wrap* creates an effective barrier between body juices and can be a lot of fun. It shouldn't be used as a condom unless absolutely necessary. But its "see through" quality makes for a wonderful body wrap for those who need extra skin protection. It is also great to use just for the fun of it.

Getting Tested

Most STD's come from viruses and bacteria and although they may be serious in nature, they are nothing to be ashamed of. Think how silly it would seem if you were ashamed of having the flu or a cold. Sex is nothing to be ashamed of and neither are infections that are transmitted sexually.

If you are sexually active you should be tested at least every six months. If you have multiple partners, get tested more frequently.

If you or your partner(s) notice any unusual discharge, pain with urination, bumps or ulcerations, get tested immediately. You can find services through the internet under "STD testing and the name of your city" or contact the Institute for Advanced Study of Human Sexuality www.iashs.edu for a referral. Also you can find services listed in your local yellow pages under Clinics, Family Planning or Health Services.

Asking for Help

Another way of protecting yourself is asking for professional help.

If you need to talk to someone about STD's, sexual relationships, prevention, risk, sexual preferences or if a family member or friend has HIV, help is out there.

You can:
- call the nearest college or university that has a human sexuality program. They can usually provide names of several clinical sexologists or sex-positive therapists in the area.
- get the names of sex-positive doctors from friends within your community.
- contact the Institute for Advanced Study of Human Sexuality www.iashs.edu for a referral.

You need to interview each one to make sure that you feel comfortable with them and that they have worked through their own issues about safer sex. You also need to watch out for the counselor whose denial system is such that they minimize the problem, rationalizing that you are at greater risk just crossing the street than contacting the any STD, including AIDS and leaving you feeling that all you need to do to be safe is to avoid sexual contact with gay or bisexual men or prostitutes.

At the other extreme are the helping professionals who are so frightened that they may suggest you stop being sexual or give up large and important aspects of your sexual behavior or lifestyle, for example anal intercourse, swinging, French kissing, relating to men on a sexual basis, S/M and open relationships.

You want a sex-positive professional who can non-judgmentally assist you.

Once you have chosen someone, you must be specific about your concerns. There is little use in spending a great deal of time on the pros and cons of condom usage when what you are really worried about is communication about safe sex. Likewise, sexual communication skills are premature if you feel that sex equals death or that sperm is toxic. With your therapist, you can set realistic goals, objectives and a time frame to work from.

Your therapist will be assisting you to:
- look at the emotional feelings that emerge for you between each session
- identify sex-negative messages and replace them with positive and reaffirming ones
- validate your right to be sexual, even in the age of AIDS
- notice resistance on an emotional level and discover ways of working through your resistance
- clarify sexual preferences

CHAPTER FIVE: JUST FOR TEENS

*This chapter was written by **Loretta Haroian, Ph.D.** Formally the world's leading expert on childhood and adolescent sexuality. Dr. Haroian gave her genius in understanding how children and adolescents actually learn about sex. Her words are as powerful and appropriate today as the day she wrote them.*

*I*f you are a teen and reading this, remember it's often hard to take adult warnings seriously in your teens because you feel invincible. However, the risks are real and you need to make some important decisions about sex and drugs. STD's, including HIV/AIDS are at an all time high in your age group. That means protection either isn't being used or is not used properly.

The danger of STD's is especially problematic for teens for many reasons.
- Sexual interest, curiosity and desire are high teenage priorities.
- Even though you may be scared about STD's, your natural, normal, healthy, biological sexual drive is strong and demanding.
- Most teens have few or no resources of accurate information about STD's, risk, protection and sexual matters in general.
- Teens are reluctant to talk to any adult about their sexual activity.
- Sexual experimentation with more than one partner is common in mid to late teens.

- Many teens are also experimenting with drugs.
- Spontaneous, opportunistic sexual encounters may find you unprepared to protect yourself from pregnancy and STD's.
- Inexperience, lack of knowledge and embarrassment make it difficult to negotiate for safe sex practices.
- Teens (especially girls) are reluctant to buy, carry and use condoms.
- Many girls use no protection at all against pregnancy or STD's.
- Many girls have sex for nonsexual reasons and do whatever the boy wants because they want the boy.
- Many boys and girls think that practicing safe sex means using birth control pills.

Read and reread this book; share it with friends and refer to it often. Find a knowledgeable adult with whom you can discuss your personal sexual concerns, someone you trust enough to tell everything. If you have done something sexual you think may have placed you at risk, tell that person so they can help you put it in perspective, do the appropriate thing, and stop worrying.

If you need personal information and wish to remain anonymous, call a sex information hotline or contact the Institute for Advanced Study of Human Sexuality www.iashs.edu for a referral.

In order to know what to do about it you must:
- Determine your level of risk.
- Take responsibility for yourself.
- Practice safe sex.

If you follow these simple guidelines, you can help protect yourself from STD's:

- Know that no one cares as much about your life and health as you do.
- Don't think that you can fool yourself and sneak around these principles. You may luck out, but then again you may not.
- Don't have sex when drunk or high. Sex is its own high.
- Know that the desire, urgency and pleasure of the moment is not worth the risk of unprotected sexual intercourse. Don't be talked into unprotected sex because neither of you has condoms or because one of you says it isn't natural, doesn't feel as good, he won't love you anymore, he'll find someone else or any other excuse.
- Don't be talked into sex for nonsexual reasons. Don't believe that if you give sex because your partner wants it, s/he will like you better or longer. They might just like sex and be willing to say anything to convince you to have it.
- Don't depend on your partner to provide protection or good judgment in all sexual situations. S/he may put pressure on you when drunk or high or particularly horny. You need the courage to stand firm even if you are begged or threatened.
- Know that many young people reserve sexual intercourse for marriage or a committed relationship.
- Know that most of the sexual activities called petting, including mutual masturbation to climax, are safe and satisfying.

You have the right to be sexual and to know everything you want or need to know about sex. The consequences of sex can change your life and you accept the responsibilities when you decide to engage in sex. The rewards of sex enhance the quality of life and are enhanced when you make responsible decisions and choices. Remember the three R's of sex: **Rights, Responsibilities and Rewards**.

CHAPTER SIX: PLEASURE

*T*he brain is the most powerful sexual organ, however it's your mind that runs the show. If your mind is full of negative beliefs about sex, it is difficult to experience sexual pleasure.

Negative beliefs about sex may cause you to put a limitation on the amount of pleasure you will allow yourself to have in general, and with sex in particular. This limitation can cause you to be unhealthy – physically, mentally and emotionally, as well as sexually.

When you look back in history and see where negative beliefs about sex and pleasure originate, you can see that these beliefs are not based in logic, nature or truth but in fear and control – parents, government, society, religion. Creating natural and healthy beliefs, regarding your body and your sexuality, are imperative to pleasure and your health in general.

Establish Beliefs about Sexuality

Core beliefs are the central or most important beliefs you have. All of your beliefs are based on core beliefs. You can create a positive impact on your sexual attitude and behaviors by starting with a willingness to acknowledge and accept these core beliefs about your sexuality.

Core beliefs about sexuality are:
- Your sexuality is an integral part of who you are.
- You own your sexuality – no one can take it from you.
- It is healthy for your body to give and receive pleasure.

Defining and Changing Beliefs about Sex and Pleasure

Sexual pleasure is not taught in school and it usually not talked about at home. Most attitudes about sex, which stem from the Victorian age, are still with you.

You must first look at your beliefs about your own sexuality in order to have more sexual pleasure. Do you believe sex is sacred? Wonderful? Sinful? Disgusting? Natural? Beautiful? Do you enjoy sex or do you feel guilty? Do you have sex for pleasure or out of obligation?

The first step to changing any negative sexual beliefs is understanding that they are just that - beliefs. Beliefs are based on information that comes into the mind from family, friends, religion, society and the media. Taking charge of what is *in* your mind is your job and the key to your freedom.

Examine your beliefs:
1. Make a list of all your beliefs about sex, positive and negative. Next to the belief, write down where the belief originated.
2. Ask yourself: Does this belief empower me? Does it really represent who I am and what I want? Does it give me pleasure?
3. If you answered "no" to any of the questions, rewrite a new belief.

Here is an example. Say you want to talk 'dirty' when having sex because you think it might be exciting but you have a belief that says, "If I talk 'dirty' my partner will think I'm cheap and leave me." Where did this belief come from? Catholic school? Pier groups? A movie from the 1950's? This belief came into your mind from an outside source. It definitely does not empower you. It does not represent who you are and what you want. And, it certainly does not give you pleasure. You can rewrite it, say it out loud and instill a more positive and pleasurable belief in your minds. For example, a positive belief would be: "Talking 'dirty' is hot. It turns me on and when I get turned on my partner gets turned on."

Ingredients for Sexual Pleasure

The basic ingredients for sexual pleasure come from within you. They do not involve a partner. The more you know, love and please yourself the more sexual pleasure you will be able to enjoy in general.

These core ingredients are:
- Self-knowledge
- Self-love
- Self-image
- Self-pleasure

Let's look at these individually and see what you can do to enhance these components of your lives in order to create more sexual pleasure.

Self-Knowledge

Self-Knowledge is about knowing your body, how to take care of it, and how to identify its needs, wants and pleasures. Taking time and getting to know how your body operates is the key for creating maximum pleasure. What gives you energy? What makes you happy? What are your hot spots (places on your body that give you pleasure)?

Getting to know yourself will empower you and it's also fun.

Here are a few ideas on how you can get to know your sensual and sexual self:

- What do you love, don't particularly like and are neutral about sexually?
- What turns you on visually, what turns you off?
- What sounds or words do you like to make or hear when you are being sexual?
- What smells get you excited, which ones turn you off?
- What tastes are yummy when you are sexual, what doesn't taste good?
- What flavors (foods, lotions, oils) would you enjoy using to enhance smell and taste?
- How do you like being touched? What is too hard and too soft?
- Where do you like being touched? You can explore your entire body and find all the hot spots.
- What kind of movement do you like? What is too fast and too slow?
- How do you want your partner to look, smell and taste?
- Do you like to share your self-pleasure?
- When do you like to fantasize (daydream) about sex?
- What types of fantasies turn you on?
- Do you like to experiment with different kinds of fantasies?
- Do you like to share fantasies?
- Do you like to act out some fantasies?
- Who would you share sex fantasies with?
- Who wouldn't you share sex fantasies with?

Exercises for Self-Exploration

- **Keep a journal and/or scrapbook.** Journals are great for keeping the answers to your self-knowledge questions and to keep track of feelings, beliefs, attitudes and adventures. Journals are also great for checking in on how you feel and how your feelings, beliefs, likes and dislikes may be changing. Journals can be like diaries or outrageous creations—a box filled with jotted down thoughts, mementos of sexual experiences, stories, pictures and photos. It's your journal; therefore you can be as creative as you want.

- **Learn to be your own best sexual partner.** Do you please yourself? Do you allow enough time to be completely satisfied? Are you loving and tender? Are you hot and wild? Do you take excellent care of yourself?

- **Learn to be a great communicator.** A basic component of good sex is good communication. In order to clearly communicate your sexual concerns, needs and desires, you must first know what they are. Self-pleasuring is a great way to discover the responses of your own body.

- **Learning how you breathe.** Breathing is a naturally occurring event in the body; however, awareness and control of the rate and rhythm of your breath is not. Learning to become aware and in control of your breathing is a powerful tool in learning to relax, reducing stress and anxiety. Learning how to control your breathing also helps your body to function at an optimal level, and is great for prolonging, increasing and maintaining sexual pleasure and health. Deep breathing helps purify and oxygenate your blood.

- **Practicing abdominal breathing.** Also known as diaphragmatic or pelvic breathing helps develop relaxed breathing in the pelvic region. You can begin by lying on the floor or a bed with arms at your side and legs uncrossed. A small pillow under your head or neck and under your knees might make you more comfortable. Once comfortable, you can close your eyes and begin breathing slowly and quietly, inhaling through the nose and exhaling through the mouth. Imagine the air slowly filling the abdomen. Placing one hand lightly on your lower abdomen, you can concentrate on the movement of your abdomen as you breathe. Your hand is being pushed upwards by the abdomen as you inhale, and, as you exhale, you can push down gently on the abdomen to push your breath out further than you normally do. Exhale twice as slowly as you inhale, making sure you exhale fully. Pausing after each exhalation, and taking your time. When you do this a few times you notice how relaxed and yet energized you feel.

- **Practicing Kegel exercises.** These are a must for optimal sexual pleasure. Kegel exercises are designed to strengthen and give you voluntary control over a muscle called the pubococcygeus muscle or P.C. for short. This muscle is the support muscle for the genitals in both men and women. There is a definite correlation between good tone in the P.C. muscle and orgasmic intensity. This exercises increases blood circulation in your genital area and increases your awareness of genital sensations. "Kegels" will also add to your sexual responsiveness and increase control over your orgasms. For women who have sex with men, it helps them grip the penis and increase pleasure for both partners. It also aids in restoring vaginal muscle tone following childbirth. You can find your P.C. muscle, when you need to urinate. Starting and stopping the flow of urine is the job of the P.C. muscle. Practicing stopping and staring the flow, without moving your legs together, will strengthen that muscle. Sometimes it takes time to get this down, but if you keep practicing you will get it. Once you can stop and start at will, you will know the feeling of tightening these muscles. Your next step is to practice, when you are not urinating. You can do slow Kegels by tightening your P.C. muscle and holding it, as you did when you stopped the flow of urine, for a slow count of 3. Then relax the muscle. Practice quick Kegels by tightening and relaxing the P.C. muscle as rapidly as possible.

- **Sensuous bathing.** Taking a sensuous bath or shower to experience touching and exploring your body is an excellent way to increase personal sensory awareness and discover new erotic sensations. What makes you feel good? You can explore your entire body – touch, stroke, massage and caress.

- **Learn to use fantasy.** While most people fantasize frequently, you, most likely, won't have the time, energy, ability or the desire to act out most of what you fantasize about. This is normal. Many people forget that fantasy is not reality and feel guilty if their sexual fantasies are nontraditional, politically incorrect or otherwise "inappropriate." While fantasies can't force you to do things you don't want to do, you can use fantasies to empower action. Therefore, it is extremely important to create and explore fantasies.

Fantasies are:
- a great way to get turned on
- something you can do for yourself, by yourself
- fun to verbalize
- enriching to your sex life
- fun to share with the right partner
- safe
- innocent
- fun to act out

Fantasies are something you can have while…
- talking on the phone
- grocery shopping
- working in the garden
- having sex
- looking at porn
- eating
- sleeping
- bathing
- reading this book

Acting out your fantasies would make you:
- happy
- exhausted
- disappointed
- embarrassed
- break the law
- mortified
- hurt yourself and others
- liberated
- a contortionist

Your sexual fantasies may sometimes involve:
- being seduced
- getting fucked
- fucking
- animals
- oral sex
- anal sex
- teasing
- being raped
- feet
- group sex
- getting spanked
- spanking
- being in love
- fisting
- children
- men
- women
- bondage
- watching others have sex

Self-Love

Self-love includes self-respect, self-esteem (your opinion of yourself), self-worth (how much you value yourself) and self-protection (caring about yourself and protecting yourself from pain and harm).

A sex positive attitude is built on self-love and self-respect. Loving and respecting yourself leads to happiness, health and success, as well as loving and respecting others.

Loving yourself also means taking responsibility for your actions and protecting yourself from harm.

Acting in a kind, loving, respectful and responsible

manner toward yourself sends a very powerful message to your subconscious that you are worthwhile. This positive message about who you are, directly affects your beliefs and, of course, your sexual behavior and sexual choices.

Keys steps to self-love:
- Take care of yourself, physically, mentally and emotionally. This includes plenty of pampering.
- Choose sex partners that are positive, kind, gentle, loving and supportive.
- Trust in the frailty of humanity and always protect yourself from STD's.

Again with self-love, your beliefs play a vital role. You must believe that you are lovable, worthwhile and someone who deserves respect.

Unconditional self-love insures that you will pick a partner that will give you the same respect and love and not settle for anything less than what you give yourself.

Self-Image

Your self-image is how you see yourself. This image may or may not be based in reality. Working on establishing powerful core beliefs about your self is the first step to a great self-image.

Your body image plays a critical part in your pleasure, especially in sexual pleasure. How you see yourself, whether it is accurate or not, usually will determine how you are sexually (especially with a partner) and how much pleasure you allow yourself to have.

You may know someone with a great body who thinks they are too fat or a beautiful woman who believes she is ugly.

And, you may know someone who is neither beautiful nor fit and that person may be happy with themselves and their looks.

Here are some suggestions for you to change your body image:

- Work on core beliefs (see *Establish Core Beliefs*)
- Start with the body you have - love it, pamper it and make it into the healthiest, fittest body you possibly can.
- Make a list of what you like and don't like about your body. Change what you can and accept and love what you can't.
- Visualize yourself as a unique work of art with each little line on your face or physical imperfection adding to that uniqueness.

Establish Core Beliefs

Establish core beliefs by writing them down and affirming them by saying them out loud. Post it notes work well for recording your new beliefs because you can attach them to your bathroom mirror or computer screen as a reminder.

Some great core beliefs are:

- I am positive, kind, gentle, loving, supportive and respectful.
- I treat myself, others and all of life with kindness, love and respect.
- My body is my temple and I treat it with the utmost care and respect and I require that same treatment from others.

- I have unlimited power and energy.
- I can be, do or have anything I want.
- I look for the good in everything that happens to me.
- I am part of everything that is good and worthwhile.

Sexual Self-Pleasure

It is important to give yourself sensual and sexual pleasure. Taking time for yourself and pampering yourself builds your capacity for pleasure and increases your ability to receive pleasure. Allowing your body to enjoy heightened sexual pleasure helps you to progressively go beyond your pleasure limitations.

Using your senses, you can experience seeing, hearing, smelling, tasting and touching in a sexual and pleasurable way. While you are doing this you can allow your imagination to run wild with internal sexual images, sounds, smells, tastes and touch.

In order to do this, it is important for you to create a special time and safe space to explore your body and learn to give yourself pleasure. You need to make "pleasure appointments" with yourself. An hour a day is optimal but anytime you have, even small increments of time – 10 or 15 minutes, several times a day is great.

Some ideas on scheduling pleasure time are:
- Make taking time for yourself a priority.
- Turn off phones, computers, or do anything else that interrupts your enjoyment.
- Make a place that is sexy, sensual, soft, and quiet.
- Discover books, pictures, music textures, and/or smells that are especially sensuous, enjoyable, and erotic and be willing to add them to your environment.

Do things for yourself that please your outer senses:
- sight (movies, pictures, soft lighting, etc.)
- hearing (music, etc.)
- smell (scented candles, flowers, etc.)
- taste (food, your own body, etc.)
- touch (self-massage, textures, lotions, etc.)

Do things that please your inner senses:
- reading uses internal visual and auditory senses
- fantasy uses your imagination and can draw on all five senses: internally see, hear, smell, taste and touch your fantasies.
- sensual dancing awakens internal passions. Allowing your body to feel the music deep inside. Letting the music move you and the movement, massage you.

Explore new ways to:
- Reach sexual fulfillment
- Lengthen and intensify orgasms
- Discover the erotic potential of your entire body
- Discover what turns you on and what turns you off
- Playing with multiple orgasm potential (yes, even for men! –see exercises under Expanding your Enjoyment.)

Sexual self-pleasure is …
- a wonderful gift you can give yourself
- a great way to have a quick orgasm(s)
- self-loving
- a great tension reliever
- sexually liberating
- a great way to learn about your body

Advanced Self-Pleasuring

- Use all five internal and external senses. The more senses you use, the more intense your experience will be and the more pleasure you will have.
- Include whole-body touching. Work out from the genitals, spreading the sexual energy throughout the whole body.
- Incorporate pelvic breathing. It may be awkward at first, but you will see how it affects your sexual response, the strength of your orgasms and ejaculations.
- Contract and release your P.C. (Kegel) muscles, Also incorporate pelvic thrusting to add to the intensity.
- Concentrate on your pelvis. What happens when you relax it? What happens when you lift and contract it? How does your pelvis feel when you contract your anus? What happens when you contract your P.C. (Kegel) muscles? Do these pelvic movements heighten arousal? Prolong orgasmic plateau? Make the clitoris more sensitive, the penis harder?

Expanding your Enjoyment

Here are some ways to expand the enjoyment of self-pleasure. These exercises can assist you in learning how your body feels at the different stages of arousal and show you how to use this information to increase sexual pleasure.

More self-pleasure exercises:
- Build orgasms.
- Prolong orgasms
- Have multiple orgasms
- Experience orgasms outside the genitals

Build Orgasms

Self-pleasure until you feel your breathing increase, until you feel like going very fast, and/or until you experience wanting to thrust your pelvis. Then you can stop and experience these feelings for a while. Learn to build up sexual pleasure, and then let it subside. Become aware of the feelings, relax a little, and then continue. Don't aim for an orgasm.

You can take a short break, one or two minutes, and then begin again using light stroking and incorporate Kegels. When there is sufficient lubrication in the vagina, or when you notice a secretion from the penis, you can take a few moments to smell and taste your own secretions. It's perfectly okay to like your own body juices. The smell, taste and feel of your own juices may make you hotter.

Continue self-pleasuring until you get to the edge of climax and then stop, slow down and breathe. After you have brought yourself to the edge several times you may wish to rest, continue or try something else. Slowly building orgasms creates more intensity, more control and more pleasure.

Prolong Orgasms

Watching how your body responds as you near climax can help you prolong orgasm.

Do you hold your breath? Do you throw your head back? Do you tense and contract your pelvis and anal sphincter? If a male, do your testicles rise up close to the penis just before ejaculation? Do you hold your testicles up to ejaculate faster? These are very common elements most men experience in the pre-orgasmic stage of sex.

To intensify this plateau, you can experiment with changing your regular pattern.

Ways to change your patterns:
- If you tend to hold your breath just before orgasm, you can try slow, deep breathing instead.
- If your neck is tensing and you want to throw it back, you can concentrate on relaxing your neck muscles and not throwing your head back.
- If you tend to lift your pelvis and/or contract your anus, you can try relaxing or even pushing down on the floor of your pelvis. You can try pushing down with your anal sphincter muscle as though you wished to defecate.
- If a male, you can experiment with relaxing your testicles. If you notice they are rising and circling your scrotum, you can gently pull them down. You might even want to hold them down for a while. You can repeat this many times to prolong sexual pleasure.
- Remember you can also stop, change positions and techniques to prolong the process of orgasm.

Multiple Orgasms

Sometimes when you change your usual pattern of having an orgasm that the intensity and duration of orgasm increases dramatically.

Many people, especially men, assume that they are not multi-orgasmic. Often they have not tried continuing sexual activity after initial orgasm. When using the techniques described above, you may find that with duration of orgasm comes the desire and ability to have more sexual activity. This makes sense because the better it feels the more you will want to do it. Men often find that if they maintain an erection this increases their sexual intensity and that enhances the possibility of having multiple orgasms.

Sexual self-pleasure is a particularly good place to become experienced at these techniques. In addition, you might want to talk with your partner or friends. Teach them some of the ways you are learning to have a better time and ask how they make their orgasms stronger and/or better.

Orgasms Outside the Genitals

Many rely entirely on their genitals for sexual gratification (this is especially true for men). However, it is often possible to have orgasms in other parts of the body that are sometimes as enjoyable, exciting and powerful as genital ones. This fact is well known to those who have lost their genital functioning for various reasons, and have had to look elsewhere on their bodies for orgasmic satisfaction. In fact, some adults who have lost all genital sensation due to spinal chord injuries report that the newly discovered and developed erotic parts of their bodies create orgasms more powerful and satisfying than any they can remember before their injury.

Learning to have orgasms in non-genital parts of the body may be easy for you or may seem impossible. However, you can learn to increase and intensify the erotic potential and sexual response of other parts of your body. Having this option is important in creating even more pleasure and, in addition, is another way of having safer sex.

A side benefit of increasing your non-genital sexual potential is that you can have a wonderful time masturbating in social situations which otherwise would be boring, unpleasant or wasted time. You just need to be careful not to start moaning and groaning inappropriately!

To start exploring and developing non-genital orgasms, it is useful to remember that you invalidate what you are experiencing sexually in three different ways:

Ways you may invalidate what you are experiencing:
- By comparing your experience to what others are experiencing. "S/he seems to be enjoying this more than I am. I must be doing it wrong."
- By comparing your experience to past experiences. "I'm not getting aroused as quickly as when I did, therefore something is wrong."
- By comparing your experience to your expectation. "I thought I'd be having orgasms every time I squeezed my nipples hard. What am I doing wrong?"

You need to forget about what you used to think was true about you, and your orgasms, and be willing to experience something new. You may just surprise yourself. Experiment any way you want to.

Below are some guidelines that others have found very useful in developing new orgasmic potential:
- Allow time. First you need to find a time when you can spend longer than you usually do for your "private time," maybe a couple of hours or the whole morning, afternoon or night.
- Set the stage. You may want to get some new things for your erotic enjoyment - satin sheets, candles, perfume, incense, feathers, oils, erotic porn, stirring music. All the elements in your environment should be an erotic delight for you.
- Wake up your entire body. You may enjoy taking a slow bath or shower, really enjoying feeling your entire body as you bathe. Do sensory exercises, dance, yoga or anything else that feels good to you.

Now you are ready to lay back, relax, breathe and take your time!

- fantasize
- breathe slowly
- do Kegels
- stroke and caress your body
- explore your ears, squeeze your nipples, play with your hair
- feel the skin between your toes, in your arm pits, under your chin, over your lips (taking your time)
- slowly move your finger tips over your body very lightly
- breathe, enjoy
- find a non-genital part of your body that feels especially good
- increase your stroking and pressure there
- find another place and yet another
- intensify the Kegels, breathing, pressure and fantasies
- continue at a comfortable pace playing, experimenting, pleasuring your body; vary the speed and intensity of your breath, Kegels, fantasies, touching, stroking, caressing, petting, pinching, pulling, tugging, slapping, tapping.

You mustn't get caught up in searching for an orgasm. This is supposed to be pleasurable. If you do begin to have an orgasm, you can stop it, slow it down or let it happen but you don't have to stop pleasuring yourself. Remember, exploring and pleasure are the goals.

When you do have an orgasm, you may find the it continues beyond initial spasms, grows stronger, turns into multiple orgasms or fizzles quickly. If you don't have an orgasm during this exploring, you don't have to worry because the goal is to have fun and increase sensory awareness.

Your body is the canvas, your breath is the paint, your mind the brush and you are the artist!

Playing with Toys and Lubes

Adding toys and lubricants (lubes) to your sex play can be a lot of fun.

Dildos (fake cocks), vibrators (in all shapes and sizes), butt plugs, vibrating cock rings are just some of the products you can play with. These and other fun products can be purchased online from a variety of websites. Check with the Institute for Advanced Study of Human Sexuality's webpage www.iashs.edu for recommended products and links.

Water-based lubes are great for self-pleasuring and toy play without the clean up mess like you can get with silicone. Water-based lubes usually come in different thicknesses - liquids and gel, depending on the feel you prefer.

Flavored lubes are great for oral sex. Using them with a condom or dam really makes latex delicious. These succulents can also be used on any and all parts of the body to increase pleasure. Succulents come in many flavors - watermelon, cherry, banana, mango, just to name a few. YUM!

Sharing Pleasure with Others

Now that you know how to protect yourself by practicing safe sex and how to please yourself by knowing your own body intimately and becoming your own best lover, you may want to share your sexuality and pleasure with an incredible, deserving and loving partner.

Communicating about Protection

Communicating with your partner is the best way to insure that you have a pleasurable sexual experience and that you protect yourself from exposure to STD's.

It is a lot easier to make decisions at a safe, non-sexual time than in the heat of passion. A great start for a safe, sexual and intimate relationship is thinking about what might happen in advance, knowing what you want to do and what you don't want to do, and understanding how to communicate this to your partner(s).

You may fear a loss of spontaneity and freedom if you have to practice safe sex. However, while you may think you are spontaneous, you may actually be in a rut. Do you have sex at the same time of day or night, using the same activities, taking the same positions, making the same sounds, and using the same sexual toys and products? If the answer is yes, instead of feeling a loss of spontaneity you may actually be experiencing loss of familiar behavior.

Practicing safe sex forces you to be creative and this creativity can get you out of any rut and can lead to more erotic pleasure.

If you are involved in a committed relationship you can tell your partner that your desire to use protection is based on your growing awareness that humans do make errors in judgment and therefore you are willing to place the burden of responsibly for yourself on yourself, and not place that responsibility on him or her.

Safe sex check list

It's helpful for you to make a detailed list of what you will do when having sex, what you absolutely won't do and what is up for negotiation. A YES, NO and MAYBE list.

First, it may be a good practice to share your list with someone you don't intend to be sexual with. Talking about why you feel the way you do, practicing negotiating what the two of you could do if you were going to be sexual. This will help you determine if there are parts of the list that are easier to negotiate than others?

Next, you can share this list with someone you want to be sexual with, before the clothes come off.

The Yes/No Exercise

Choose a partner who has made their own YES, NO and MAYBE list - anyone who is adventurous and into improving their safe sex communication skills. A major purpose of the exercise is to strengthen your ability to hold to your resolve under all kinds of conditions.

- Pick something from your YES list.
- Your partner picks something from their NO list.
- Don't tell each other what was picked.
- Stand face-to-face.
- For two minutes, try to convince your partner to do what you feel is okay just by saying yes while your partner tries to convince you not to do what they don't want to do just by saying no.
- You can look menacing or irresistible, BUT you can only say one word: YES, and your partner can only say NO.
- Reverse roles. You pick from your NO list and your partner picks something from their YES list.
- Share with your feelings about the exercise with each other. It may be empowering to realize that "No!" is a complete statement!

Communication Exercise

Even in the best relationships, there are differences of opinion. This is a great exercise whether the difference of opinion is about practicing safe sex or anything else. The purpose of this exercise is to provide each partner an open "safe" space in which to express his or her feelings (good or bad) about something, and to provide the assurance that each has been heard.

- Schedule time so there are no interruptions.
- One person talks for 5 minutes and the other listens.
- The talker uses "I" statements such as, "I feel…" "I want…"   "I am…" and sticks to their feelings and their needs.
- The talker does not use "You" statements such as, "You always…" "You feel…" "You need…"   This is not about assumptions or blame.
- The listener may not interrupt except to ask for clarification, for example, "Could you be more specific."
- After the talker is finished, the listener says "Thank you."
- The listener may take notes in order to be accurate when responding. For example, "I heard you say. . . is that what you said?"
- The listener may respond immediately or within 24 hours.
- The listener gets to have 5 minutes to respond. Using "I" statements about his or her feelings and needs.

Some people enjoy getting and giving response immediately after the exercise while some find it helpful to wait at least twenty-four hours before responding. You can negotiate with your partner before the exercise as to when to give or get response.

Erotic and Intimate Sex

Having sex in a close, personal and loving relationship for mutual excitement and pleasure is erotic and intimate. Sex that is based solely on performance, penetration and release is usually not about eroticism or intimacy. Although "quickies" certainly have their place, and may be about mutual pleasure, this section is dedicated to taking your time, building up excitement and enjoying your sexuality with your partners(s).

When your actions are intended to arouse or evoke sexual desire in yourself and/or in someone else, you are being erotic. Turning someone on sexually means to fill that person with pleasure, energy and excitement in the same way you were filled with pleasure, energy and excitement during your own self-pleasuring.

In the beginning of a relationship, turning someone on or getting turned on seems to come naturally. However, as the relationship continues sometimes sex becomes stale.

Here are just a few things you can do things to evoke newness in the relationship and keep sex hot:
- undress your partner, slowly and intentionally, paying attention to every inch of his or her body
- undress for your partner, slowly and intentionally, watching your partner watch you
- dance for your partner and dance together
- watch videos together
- pleasure yourself as your partner watches

- pleasure your partner and look into his or her eyes
- create atmosphere -candles, soft music, scents, etc.
- breathe in your partners scents, let your partner know how much you enjoy their scent
- engage in love talk, whisper, sigh, talk "dirty"
- sensually describe your fantasies, maybe act out a few
- listen carefully as your partner talks about his or her fantasies
- play with new toys and lubes
- massage your partner
- bathe your partner

You can continue to add to this list. You can do whatever looks, smells, tastes, sounds and feels good that is sexy and safe. You can allow yourself to be creative and use your imagination! You can most definitely have fun!

Creating More Intimacy and Mutual Pleasure
You don't want to rely on your partner(s) to know more about your body and your pleasure than you do. You know your body intimately though self-pleasuring, now its time to share that wealth of information. Also, you don't want to assume that you know your partner(s) likes and dislikes based on your own body. Everyone is different and you can let your partner know what makes you hot and find out what makes your partner hot. The following exercises are to help you learn more about your partner's body and for them to learn more about yours. Also, you can use these exercise to reach a new level of intimacy, communication and pleasure.

Sharing Sexual Self-Pleasuring

Although most people pleasure themselves sexually, most have been taught to be secretive about it. However, if you talk with others who are willing to share their experience, you often feel better about doing it and learn many new ways to pleasure yourself. You can share the information you have learned about your self-pleasuring and experimentation and find out how other people feel about theirs. This can be in a sexual or non-sexual context with your spouse, lover, friend, or support group.

Try out the following exercise:

Choose a partner with whom to share information about self-pleasuring patterns. The questions below will help clarify your own views and attitudes as well as give you an opportunity to understand another point of view. Decide who will ask the question first and who will answer. When finished, change roles.

Ask each other:
- When is the earliest self-pleasuring you can remember?
- When did you first associate self-pleasuring with the term masturbation?
- How did you learn to self-pleasure? (self-discovery, friend, etc.)
- When did you have your first conversation about self-pleasure?
- How did you feel about self-pleasuring as a teenager?
- How do you feel about self-pleasuring now?
- How do you self-pleasure? Do you ever try different ways?
- Do you use toys and/or lubes?

Sharing sexual self-pleasuring is also an ideal way for you to show your partner(s) the kind of touching, stroking and timing you like and all the parts of your body that help to intensify your pleasure.

Sharing Fantasies

Fantasies are wonderful. Sharing fantasies with a partner can be very hot and very intimate.

Sharing fantasies is a powerful tool to:
- Define and clarify your feelings
- Enrich your sexual experiences together
- Enhance intimacy and trust

You can play with fantasies with your partner(s) and share the fantasy exercises from the self-pleasure section or make up some new ones.

Phone Sex

Phone sex is an excellent way to share fantasies. Keep in mind that this refers to consensual behavior and is not to be confused with illegal, nonconsensual, harassing and obscene phone calls. Consensually listening to someone's hot, steamy, sexy voice on the other end of the telephone while you are getting off is not a new phenomenon. However, it has never been as widespread as it is today, nor have there been the wide range of commercial services that are currently available.

While having phone sex, you can add to the intensity by consciously contracting and releasing your P.C. (Kegel) muscles. You can incorporate using protection in a very erotic and pleasurable way in your fantasies. Also, you can use your "bedroom voice" - hot, sultry, sexy!

Tips for hot, phone sex:

- Read your favorite erotic literature to your partner, imagine your lover playing with your body as you're doing this.
- Call your lover at a time they can't respond adequately (like when they are at work) and tell them, in as much graphic detail as possible, the parts of their body that drive you wild with desire, and why.
- Describe, in detail, your favorite fantasies.
- Plan an uninhibited time together and you can be very detailed about what you want to do to your partner and what you want your partner to do to you.
- Give your lover detailed sexy instructions on self-pleasuring, oral sex and anything else that makes your blood boil.
- Pretend to be a new fantasy lover and describe yourself, and what you would like to do to them, if they would only be willing to meet you right now in some dark secluded place!
- While you and your partner are mutually self-pleasuring, you can imagine that your hand is your partner's hand, and tell your partner how it feels.
- During a long, slow sensuous bath, you can call your lover and tell him or her how incredible your body feels in the hot water and what you would like him or her to be doing to you right now.
- Plan for your lover to call you at a specific time and tell your lover how you want her or him dressed or undressed.
- Leave a sexually explicit message on your lover's answering machine when you are sure they're the only one who will receive it.

- Together you can call one of the sexually explicit phone services that are in abundance right now, and get ideas on how to spice up your own phone fantasy play.
- If you are into group sex, you could consider making conference calls.

The possibilities are only as limited as your imagination. You can give yourself permission to be imaginative, experimental and outrageous.

You can get consent from anyone you would like to call and negotiate the parameter of your calls by asking the following questions:

- Is it okay to phone in the middle of the night?
- Can I call you at work?
- Are there any fantasies that would be upsetting to you?
- What fantasies turn you on the most?

Bathing with your Partner

Bathing with a partner is sensuous and erotic. As you bathe your partner let each step of the process teach you something new about them.

Here are a few tips that you can do before your partner arrives to make bathing together more adventurous and enjoyable:

- Create atmosphere. Remove from sight everything possible that says, "This is a bathroom."
- Flowers, candles and music do wonders for transforming a bath into a magical experience. Drape lush towels or beautiful fabric over the toilet.

- Take down the shower curtain or remove the sliding doors from a tub for a bath, to create more room and enhance the atmosphere.

In the tub, one way you can bathe your partner's upper body is to sit behind them so that his or her back rests upon your chest. Then you can reach around his or her body to wash and explore. This can be a very nurturing experience.

When it is your turn to be bathed, give yourself permission to relax and be taken care of.

Sensuous Erotic Massage

Massage is all about pleasure. Whether you are massaging or being massaged, you can get into the sensual nature of the experience. If you are giving the massage, cherish the individual you are playing with.

Here are a few things you can try:
- experiment with different kinds of strokes, and different combinations
- vary pressure, using your fingertips, hands, arms, elbows, eyelashes, chest - your entire body
- get feedback on pressure and types of touch, ask your partner what they like and don't like.
- incorporate whatever toys you may have around, discover the ones that your partner enjoys the most and the ones that are the most fun for you to use
- vary lubrication – oil, warmed oil, cream and savoring the contrast
- be creative and enjoy the pleasure of giving pleasure

Erotic Massage and Body Mapping

This erotic massage serves two purposes. One, you

get to give and receive pleasure and two, to you get to create an erotic map, with your partner, of your body and your partner's body.

- Choose who will receive the first massage. Partner **A** and **B**. Say partner **A** goes first.
- Set aside 30 minutes for each massage
- For the purpose of this exercise let this be an erotic non-sexual massage. Remember erotic means to arouse feelings of sexual desire not necessarily to act on those feelings.

The first half of the massage is entirely under partner **A**'s direction.

A will tell **B** exactly what they want and don't want:
- what kind of oil, lotion, if any, **A** prefers
- where to start: toes, shoulders, face
- the kind of pressure **A** wants
- the kind of stroking **A** wants
- when to add more oil, cream or talc
- when to move to another area
- when to change stroking
- whether or not to use feathers, etc.

The second half of the massage is entirely under the direction of partner **B**. **A** just lays back and enjoys. Interjecting only if there is something **A** absolutely doesn't like or doesn't want.

After **A**'s massage, continue to relax for another 15 minutes, or however long it takes, while partner **B** draws **A**'s body map.

On a large sheet of paper, **B** will draw an outline of a body to represent **A**'s body and do the following:

- Circle the areas where **A** were most responsive and least responsive
- Draw thick lines where **A** liked hard touch, thin lines for soft touch and short strokes for feathery touch.
- Become totally creative and detailed and have fun.
- Put drawing aside to share latter.

Now, it's time to switch. **A** gives the massage.

This time the first half of the massage is entirely under **B**'s direction. **B** will tell **A** exactly what he or she wants and doesn't want.

The second half of the massage is entirely under A's direction. This time **B** gets to lay back and enjoy.

After **B**'s massage, he or she continues to relax for another 15 minutes, or however long it takes, for **A** to draw **B**'s body map.

On a large sheet of paper, **A** will draw an outline of a body to represent **B**'s body and do the following:

- Circle the areas where **B** was most responsive and least responsive
- Draw thick lines where **B** liked hard touch, thin lines for soft touch and short strokes for feathery touch.
- Become totally creative and detailed and have fun.

When you are both are finished, share your maps and take the time to communicate about the experience:

- What did you learn from the experience?
- What did you learn about your individual sensual and erotic responses?

- What kinds of touching do each of you like the best?
- How accurate were you in drawing your partner's body map?
- How accurate did you think your partner was in drawing your map?
- Which massage was the easiest to give? To receive?
- Which was the most enjoyable, the hardest, the most relaxing?
- Which one would you like to repeat?
- Was it hard to give directions?
- Were you distracted by worrying about what your partner was thinking, feeling, or experiencing?
- Did you feel as though you were being listened to?
- Did you feel safe?   Nurtured? Pleasured?

CELEBRATE

Armed with accurate information, empowered with self-knowledge and sex positive beliefs, you can go out and enjoy your sexuality – safely and with pleasure!

APPENDIX

STUDIES ON DISCLOSURE

In the study, Sex, Lies and HIV, conducted on 665 southern California students in 1990:

- 34% of the men and 10% of the women have told lies in order to have sex. Few people actually know if they have been exposed to infections.
- 68% of the men and 59% of the women have been involved with more than one person that their current partner does not know about.
- 47% of the men and 42% of the women would understate the number of their previous partners in order to convince someone to have sex.

In 1998, a survey of Sexual Attitudes and Behavior, with 300 students at the University of Cincinnati found:

- 25.6% of men and 14.5% of the women have told lies in order to have sex.
- 10% of the men and 7.8% of the women would lie about being HIV negative, when they were not sure or never tested,
- 19.8% of the men and 17.3% of the women would not tell their partner they knew they were HIV positive.
- 75.6% of the men and 66.7% of the women, who have been sexual with more than one person at a time, did not their partners they had other partners.
- 20% of the respondents said they would never disclose a single act of infidelity.
- The majority of the students were not very concerned about contracting HIV.

In 1999, the survey of Sexual Attitudes and Behaviors at the University of Cincinnati was repeated, only this time with 637 students. The results were as follows:

- 41.5% of men and 18% of the women have told lies in order to have sex.
- 25.3% of the men and 19.7% of the women would lie about being HIV negative, when they were not sure or never tested,
- 22.4% of the men and 19% of the women would not tell their partner they knew they were HIV positive.
- 70.2% of the men and 71.0% of the women, who have been sexual with more than one person at a time, did not tell their partners they had other partners.
- 25% of the respondents said they would never disclose a single act of infidelity.
- The majority of the students were not very concerned about contracting HIV.

STUDIES ON SPERMICIDES/MICROBICIDES
In 1999, a study was conducted by the Institute for Advanced Study of Human Sexuality on three hundred and forty-nine women about STD's and protection. The results were as follows:

- 92.3% said that it was very important that women to be educated about how to protect themselves against STD's.
- Most of the women (74.5%) felt that it was very important to have information to help protect themselves against STD's
- Most of the women (77.94%) felt that women in general needed to be concerned about getting STD's from their partners but only 22.9% felt they had to

be concerned about getting STD's from their own partner and over half the women felt they were not at risk.

- Over 50% of the women said that a topical microbicide, that was effective, would be a valuable product for women in general and for them in particular.
- Over 50% of the women responding said that were willing to pay $12.00 for 12 applications.
- Over 50% said they would be willing to pay $2.00 more if the product included a buffering agent to that there would be no allergic reaction or irritation.
- 94% of the women wanted a microbicide/contraceptive product.
- Over 90% said that a topical microbicide was useful.
- 96% felt that a single application product should be provided and should cost $1.00.
- Almost 90% of the women felt that the government, in combination with foundations should pay for a microbicide product for third world countries.
- 83% of the women felt that the Institute should make a videotape on topical microbicides and also provide samples of a product that people can try. Over 50% said they would pay $10. for a video plus 6 individual applications.

GLOSSARY

Abstinence Not taking part in sexual acts. Some people include masturbation in this definition, others do not. Some people use celibacy to denote this concept, but that actually means: to not marry (i.e. vow of celibacy). Asceticism is also used, but is more of a denial of all pleasure.

AC/DC See Bisexual

Acquired Immunodeficiency Syndrome A disease caused by one of a family of viruses which break down the body's immune system leaving it open to opportunistic infections. See HIV.

AIDS See Acquired Immunodeficiency Syndrome.

Ambisexual See Bisexual.

Anal Copulation A form of sexual intercourse involving penetration of the anus by the penis. Please note that both men and women can be anally copulated. This is also called anal coitus. Slang terms include corn holing, ass fucking, Greek, and buggery.

Anal Eroticism Finding sexual enjoyment in the stimulation of one's own or a partner's anus. See ass play.

Anal-oral Sex See Analingus.

Analingus A sexual behavior involving contact between the mouth and the anus. Also called anilinctus and anal-oral sex. Slang terms include rimming, rim job, reaming and ream job.

Analinctus See Analingus.

Ano-manual Intercourse A sexual act involving placing a hand in a partner's anus. After insertion the hand is made into a fist and a thrusting motion is made.

Anal sex See Anal Copulation

Antibody A protein produced by the body to neutralize an infection. In AIDS, these antibodies are not usually effective.

Anus The opening at the lower end of the alimentary canal. The ring of muscles between the rectum and the outside of the body. Slang terms include asshole, butt hole, and bung hole.

ARC See AIDS Related Conditions.

ARV See AIDS Related Virus.

Ass See Buttocks.

Ass Fucking See Anal Copulation.

Asshole See Anus.

Asceticism See Abstinence.

Ass Play Erotic stimulation of the anus orally, digitally, manually, with a penis or other body part or device.

B & D Also written as B/D and BD. Short for bondage and discipline. Used by some to denote a mild form of sadomasochism, but no clear distinction exists. See also Sadomasochism.

Ball See Coitus.

Balls Testicles.

Basket Slang term for male sex organs.

Beating Off See Masturbation.

Beating Your Meat See Masturbation.

Beaver See Vulva.

Behind See Buttocks.

Belly Button See Navel.

Benwa Balls A sex aid consisting of small metal or plastic balls that are placed in the vagina.

Bestiality Sexual interest and/or behavior with animals. Also called Zoophilia.

Bi See Bisexual.

Big "O" See Orgasm.

Bisexual A sexual orientation where erotic and emotional attraction to both sexes exists. Slang terms include bi, versatile, to go both ways, and AC/DC.

Blood Liquid which flows through the veins and arteries of people. Contains various cells e.g. red blood cells, lymphocytes.

Blow Job See Fellatio.

Blue Balls Painful testicles resulting from prolonged sexual stimulation without ejaculation.

Bone or Boner See Erection.

Boobs See Breasts.

Bosom See Breasts.

Box See Vagina.

Brachio-proctic Intercourse See Ano-manual Intercourse.

Breasts Area of the chest surrounding the nipple. In women this area may be enlarged and is the source of milk production. Slang terms include boobs, bosom, tits, headlights, knockers, milkcans, teats, and mammaries.

Breeders The Pejorative slang term for heterosexuals.

Buggery See Anal Copulation.

Bung Hole See Anus.

Buns See Buttocks.

Bush See Pubic Hair.

Butt See Buttocks.

Butch Slang term to describe someone or something as masculine.

Butt Hole See Anus.

Buttocks The area of the body that normally makes contact with the chair when seating. An erogenous zone for some people. Slang terms include buns, rear, can, rump, nates, behind, butt, ass, duff, and fanny.

Call Girl See Prostitute.

Can See Buttocks.

Candidiasis A common yeast infection which can be an opportunistic infection associated with AIDS. Sometimes called thrush when in the mouth or throat.

Celibacy See Abstinence.

Cervix The neck of the uterus.

Chancre A sore usually associated with syphilis.

Chastity The state of not leading an immoral life.

Chlamydia A vaginal or urinary infection that can be sexually transmitted.

Clap See Gonorrhea.

Climax See Orgasm.

Clit See Clitoris.

Clitoris The only human organ the sole purpose of which appears to be pleasure. It is part of the vulva. Slang terms include clit, little man in the boat, and jewel in the lotus.

CMV See Cytomegalovirus.

Cock See Penis.

Cock Ring A device placed around the base of the penis and testicles that aids men in getting and maintaining an erection, as well as prolonging sex.

Cocksucker Sometimes used as a derisive term, but applies to anyone who engages in fellatio.

Co-factors Other infections or genetic predispositions or environmental issues that increase either the likelihood of HIV infection or the progression of the disease.

Coitus Sexual intercourse. Often used with a modifier in front to distinguish type, e.g. anal coitus, inter-femoral coitus, etc. Slang terms include fuck, hump or ball.

Come To have an orgasm and/or ejaculation. Alternate spelling of cum. See Cum.

Condom A sheath which fits over the penis. Used for birth control and prevention of sexually transmitted diseases. Slang terms include prophylactic, scum bag, French letter, rubber, skin, and contraceptive.

Contraceptive Any device or procedure to avoid pregnancy. See Condom.

Copralalia The act of talking dirty, usually in an attempt to be sexually arousing.

Coprophilia A sexual interest in feces.

Corn Holing See Anal Copulation.

Crabs A form of body lice that look like tiny crabs. Usually found in the pubic hair.

Cum See Semen.

Cunnilinctus See Cunnilingus.

Cunnilingus Sexual stimulation of the vulva with the tongue. Also spelled cunnilinctus. Slang terms are cunt lapping, eating pussy.

Cunt See Vagina.

Cunt Lapping See Cunnilingus.

Curse The See Menstruation.

Cytomegalovirus An opportunistic infection associated with AIDS, but is common and usually occurs without AIDS.

D & S Also written D/S or DS. Short for Dominance and Submission. Another term for sadomasochism. See Sadomasochism.

Detumescence The process of losing an erection, deflation of the penis.

Diaphragm A round, latex object inserted in the vagina to cover the cervix. Used as a contraceptive or as part of a risk reduction strategy.

Dick See Penis.

Diddle See Masturbation. This term is especially used to denote female masturbation.

Digital-anal Sex Erotic stimulation of the anus with a finger or fingers.

Dildo An artificial penis.

Dose A See Gonorrhea.

Douche An internal rinsing vaginally or rectally.

Drip The See Gonorrhea.

Dry Kiss Also called a social kiss. A kiss with no exchange of saliva.

Duff See Buttocks.

Dyke See Lesbian. Sometimes pejorative depending on context.

Dysfunction Not functioning or failure to function. Often used to denote sexual problems.

Eat See Oral Sex.

EBV See Epstein-Barr Virus.

Ejaculate The fluid emitted during ejaculation.

Ejaculation Process of emitting semen from the penis.

ELISA A test for HIV antibodies.

English See Sadomasochism.

Epidemic The uncontrolled spread of a disease.

Epstein-Barr Virus A common virus which can be a serious opportunistic infection when associated with AIDS. Also has been hypothesized as a co-factor for AIDS.

Erection The engorgement of the penis with blood. Can be a sign of sexual excitement. Slang terms include bone and boner.

Erogenous Zone Any area of the body that when stimulated increases sexual excitement.

Erogeny Pertaining to sexuality and sensuality.

Erotic Anything that is sexually stimulating.

Estrogen A sex hormone found in both men and women.

Exhibitionism Sexual interest in exposing one's genitals. Slang term is flash.

Fag See Male Homosexual. Often demeaning and insulting.

Faggot See Male Homosexual. Also pejorative.

Fairy See Male Homosexual. Sometimes pejorative.

Fallopian Tube See Oviduct.

Family Jewels See Testicles.

Fanny See Buttocks.

Fellatio The sexual act of stimulating a penis orally. Colloquially called a blow job, but the action is more sucking than blowing.

Female Homosexual See Lesbian.

Fetish An erotic response to an inanimate object, for example a shoe fetish. See also Partialism.

FFA Stands for Fist Fuckers of America, not Future Farmers of America. See Ano-manual Intercourse.

Fille de Joie Literally girl of joy or joy girl. See Prostitute.

Finger Fucking Moving a finger in and out of the vagina, anus, or mouth in a manner similar to how a penis would be used. See also Digital-anal Intercourse.

Fist Fucking or Fisting See Ano-manual Intercourse. This term is usually used to describe hand-anus contact, but can be used to describe hand-vagina contact. See Vaginal-manual Intercourse.

Flaccid Non-erect, soft, especially when describing a penis.

Flagellation The striking of a partner with an instrument, usually as part of a sexual act and usually striking the back and buttocks. The instrument is usually a whip, cat-of-nine-tails, quirt, etc.

Flash See Exhibitionism.

Foreplay A misnomer for any sexual activity prior to coitus.

Fornication Coitus when unmarried.

Four-letter Word Euphemism for any word that is generally thought of as vulgar or obscene.

French See Oral Sex.

French Letter See Condom.

French Kiss See Wet Kiss.

Frigging See Masturbation. This term especially used to denote female masturbation.

Fruit See Male Homosexual. Used for humor or insults.

Fuck See Coitus.

Gang Bang See Group Sex.

Gash Male slang term for vulva or vagina. Can be pejorative.

Gay Polite word to refer to homosexual males or females.

Gay Men See Male Homosexual.

Gay Related Immunodeficiency Disease An obsolete term for AIDS.

Genitalia Scientific inclusive term for external sex organs of either sex.

Give Head See Oral Sex.

Glans The head of the penis, the area covered by the foreskin in uncircumcised men.

Glory Hole A hole in a wall or partition that a man sticks his penis through. The person on the other side then anonymously orally, manually or otherwise stimulates the penis.

Go Both Ways See bisexual.

Go Down Slang for oral sex.

Golden Shower See Urophilia.

Gonads See Testicles. Also scientific term for genitals.

Gonorrhea A sexually transmitted disease. Slang terms include clap, the drip, and a dose.

Greek See Anal Copulation. May be used in a broader sense to include any form of anal eroticism.

GRID See Gay Related Immunodeficient Disease. No longer used.

Group Sex Sexual contact among more than two people simultaneously.

Hair Pie Slang term for vulva, usually used as part of phrase "eat hair pie" referring to cunnilingus.

Hand Jobs Slang term for masturbating, especially a partner.

Hard On See Erection.

Head Give See Oral Sex.

Headlights See Breasts.

Hemophilia A genetic disease where the person's blood either does not clot or clots slowly. Only found in men.

Hepatitis A liver infection. There are several types which used to be known as infectious or noninfectious. Now know as A, B, and non-A, non-B. All types are infectious and can be transmitted sexually by the exchange of bodily fluids. Safer Sex techniques also stop the spread of hepatitis.

Herpes A slang term for a vital infection of herpes simplex I or II. This infection is exemplified by the eruption of painful blisters and can be sexually transmitted. There are several other viruses in the herpes family. All can be opportunistic infections of AIDS.

Het Pejorative term in the gay subculture for heterosexual.

Heterosexual The sexual orientation or behavior involving sex between a male and a female.

HIV See Human Immunodeficiency Virus.

Ho See Prostitute.

Homo Slang derisive term for homosexual.

Homosexual, Male See Male Homosexual.

Homosexual, Female See Female Homosexual.

Honeypot Slang term for vulva or vagina.

Hooker Slang term for prostitute.

Hormone A substance secreted by the body into the blood which controls various bodily functions. Sex hormones control menstruation, libido, 'and formation of secondary sex characteristics (i.e. growth of body hair).

Horny Slang term for being desirous of sex.

Hot Slang term for a sexual turn-on, a person or thing that evokes a strong sexual response.

HTLV-III See Human T-cell Lymphotrophic Virus III.

Human Immunodeficiency Virus The virus associated with AIDS.

Human T-cell Lymphotrophic Virus III A strain of HIV.

Hump See Coitus.

Hustler Slang term for prostitute.

Hygiene Referring to keeping the body clean and healthy.

Hymen A membrane that partially covers the opening of the vagina. Broken or greatly stretched after first coitus.

Immune Capable of being exposed to a disease and not contracting it. Most immunity is temporary.

Immune System The bodily system which fights infection by other organisms.

Immuno-globulin A substance manufactured by the immune system to help fight infections.

Immuno-suppression Suppression of the immune system.

Impotence The inability to get or maintain an erection.

Infection The state which results when a disease organism invades the body.

Infibulation The practice of piercing the genitalia or nipples and the insertion of rings or bars usually for body adornment.

Inter-femoral Between the thighs, e.g. inter-femoral intercourse or rubbing the penis between a partner's thighs.

Inter-mammary Between the breasts, e.g. inter-mammary intercourse or rubbing the penis between a partner's breasts.

Intercourse Euphemism for coitus, e.g. sexual intercourse.

Intra-uterine Device A birth control device that is placed in the uterus of a woman.

Intromission The act of placing the penis inside a partner's body, i.e. vaginal intromission, anal intromission, oral intromission.

Irrumation Colloquially, the act of fucking a mouth. The mouth is stationary and the penis moves in and out during the act. See Fellatio.

IUD See Intra-uterine Device.

Jacking Off See Masturbation.

Jack Off Party A sexual event where people masturbate either themselves or each other.

Jerking Off See Masturbation.

Jilling Off Women's slang term for female masturbation.

Jism See Semen.

J/O Party See Jack Off Party.

Jockstrap A piece of male underwear that covers the man's penis and scrotum.

John Slang for a prostitute's customer.

Joint See Penis. Also slang term for marijuana cigarette.

Joy Stick See Cock.

Kaposi's Sarcoma (KS) An opportunistic infection associated with AIDS. A rare form of cancer.

Kegels A series of exercises to strengthen the pubococcygeal (P.C.) muscles which aid in the enjoyment of sex and ease in reaching orgasm.

Kinky Slang term for any nonstandard sexual behavior or desire.

Kiss Any activity which involves the juxtaposition of the lips. See Wet Kiss and Dry Kiss.

Knockers See Breasts.

KS See Kaposi's Sarcoma.

Labia Scientific term for lips of the vagina, usually used to denote the genital labia minora and labia majora.

Lactation The process of the production and excretion of milk through the nipple.

LAV See Lymphadenopathy Associated Virus.

Lavender A slang term usually used to denote homosexual activities or events.

Lay Slang for coitus.

Leather Slang for an erotic interest in leather or the sexual style of people who wear leather (i.e. S/M).

Les Slang term for lesbian.

Lesbian A female who sees herself predominately sexually and emotionally attracted to other females.

Lesser AIDS See AIDS Related Condition.

Lezzie Pejorative slang for Lesbian.

Lez Often pejorative slang for Lesbian.

Libido Sex drive or sexual interest.

Lips See Labia

Load Slang term for ejaculate, as in "shoot your load."

Love Emotional feeling of closeness for another, sometimes used as a euphemism for coitus (e.g. making love).

Lubrication The substance, either artificial or natural, that aids insertion of penis, dildo, or fingers into an orifice.

Lust The strong physical desire to have sex with somebody, usually associated with feelings of love or affection.

Lymphadenopathy A chronic condition of swollen lymph nodes.

Lymphocytes A cell that is in the blood and the lymph fluid which is part of the body's immune system. These cells are invaded by HIV.

Lymphadenopathy Associated Virus A strain of human immunodeficiency virus.

Maidenhead Polite term for hymen.

Make Love Polite term for coitus.

Making Out See Neck.

Male Homosexual A man whose primary erotic and romantic interests are in other men.

Mammaries See Breasts.

Man in the Boat See Clitoris.

Manhole See Vagina, also Anus.

Manual-vaginal Intercourse See Vaginal-manual Intercourse.

Masochism The sexual orientation where one derives sexual pleasure from receiving physical and/or psychological pain. See also Sado-masochism.

Massage The caressing and stroking of the body for sensual enjoyment or relaxation.

Masturbation The purposeful stimulation of one's genitals to produce sexual excitement and/or orgasm. Usually thought of as a practice done to oneself, but can be done to a partner (e.g. mutual masturbation). Additionally a person may masturbate in the presence of others, see Jack Off Party. Slang terms include beating off, beating your meat, jacking off, jerking off, jilling off, frigging, and diddle.

Menstruation The approximately monthly shedding of the human female's uterine lining. The menstrual cycle is the 'hormonal cycle that results in menstruation. Slang terms include the curse and a period.

Milk Cans See Breasts.

Monogamy Literally means married to one person. Colloquially used to describe any sexually exclusive relationship.

Mons Veneris Literally means "mound of Venus.' The fat pad over the pubic bone (symphysus) in the human female which is covered with pubic hair.

Mores The beliefs of someone or group concerning the rightness or wrongness of an act or action.

Motherfucker Slang derisive term.

Mucosa The lining of the mouth, vagina, rectum, urethra etc.

Muff Slang term for vulva.

Muff Diving Slang term for cunnilingus.

Naked See Nude.

Nates See Buttocks.

Navel Structure left after the umbilicus has been sloughed off after birth.

Neck To kiss and hug. Also called making out.

Nipple Structure on the breast that milk is exuded from in females, vestigal in males. Also a source of erotic enjoyment.

Nocturnal Emission An orgasm or ejaculation during sleep. Need not be at night and can occur in women. Also called a wet dream.

Nude Without clothes.

Nuts See Testicles.

Nympho See Nymphomaniac.

Nymphomaniac A female who is supposedly sexually insatiable. Pejorative.

Obscene A pejorative term used by individuals or groups to define depictions and/or descriptions of sexual activity which they feel is offensive. At present it is properly a legal term.

Onanism Withdrawal during coitus to ejaculate.

Opportunistic Infection An infection that lies dormant in the body until the immune system is seriously damaged or compromised at which point the infection overwhelms the immune system and actively emerges.

Oral Copulation See Oral Sex.

Oral-genital Contact See Oral Sex.

Oral Sex Any sexual contact between mouth and genitals. Also called oral copulation and oral-genital sex. Slang terms include French, eat, blow job and give head.

Orchis Derived from orchid. See Testicles.

Orgasm Sexual release following a buildup of neuromuscular tension. Slang terms include the big "O" and climax.

Orgy See Group Sex.

Oviduct The tube in women which conducts the egg from the ovary to the uterus.

Ovary Female organ that produces eggs and also hormones.

Ovulation Process in which the egg is released from the ovary.

Partialism An erotic response to a part of the body, for example a foot partialism.

PCP See Pneumocystitis Carinii Pneumonia.

Pecker Slang term for penis.

Peeping Tom Slang for voyeur.

Penis Male sex organ which also serves the purpose of housing the tube (urethra) that conducts both semen and urine out of the body. Slang terms include cock, joy stick. joint, prick, dick, and rod.

Peno-vaginal Intercourse Coitus. Sexual activity with the penis inside the vagina.

Period See Menstruation.

Pessary Old term for diaphragm.

Petting Includes kissing, hugging, fondling, mutual masturbation, but not coitus.

Phallus Another term for penis.

Piercing The practice of placing various rings or bars through the body for adornment and sexual excitement.

Piss Slang for urine.

Placebo An inert substance that appears to have the effect of a drug. Used in tests of drug effectiveness.

Plasma A constituent of blood.

Pleasure A feeling of happiness, delight or satisfaction.

Pneumocystis Carinii Pneumonia An opportunistic infection related to AIDS.

Porn See Pornography.

Pornography Derogatory term used to describe sexually explicit material.

Pot Slang for marijuana.

Pox Slang for syphilis, once called great pox to differentiate it from small pox.

Prick See Penis.

Privates Euphemism for genitalia.

Promiscuous An imprecise, pejorative term related to having many sexual partners.

Prophylactic Any treatment or procedure done to avoid disease. See Condom.

Prostate A gland that surrounds the urethra at the base of the bladder in males which, during ejaculation, discharges the greater part of the semen. An erogenous zone for many men.

Prostitute Anyone who agrees to participate in sexual acts for money.

Prude A person who is overly modest or proper.

Prurient Literally means itching. Refers to a purportedly unhealthy interest in sexuality.

Puberty The process where a child develops adult sexual characteristics.

Pubic Hair Hair growth around the genitals, first appears during puberty.

Pubis Another term for the pubic area.

Pussy Slang for vagina.

Queen A homosexual man who is effeminate. Can be camp humor or term of derision.

Queer Pejorative term for homosexual.

Quickie A sexual interaction that is of short duration.

Quiff See Vagina.

Quim See Vagina.

Randy Slang term for being desirous of sex.

Rape The coerced or forced participation in sexual acts.

Ream Job See Analingus.

Reaming See Analingus.

Rear See Buttocks.

Rear Entry Coitus where intromission takes place from behind.

Rim Job See Analingus.

Rimming See Analingus.

Rod See Penis.

Rubber See Condom.

Rubber Lovers People with a fetish for latex of all sorts including rubber garments.

Rugae Technical term for the folds of tissue or ridges of the vagina.

Rump See Buttocks.

S & M Also written S/M, SM, and S-M. Slang term for sadism and masochism. though used as slave/master also. See Sadomasochism.

Sack See Scrotum.

Sadism Sexual orientation or behavior where the participant obtains erotic enjoyment from inflicting physical or psychological pain on their sexual partner.

Sadomasochism A sexual orientation and/or behavior where erotic enjoyment is obtained by giving or receiving physical or psychological pain. Slang terms include S/M, S & M, B/D, D/S and English.

Safe Sex A system of safeguards that are designed to reduce the risk of contracting HIV or other STD's.

Saliva The clear water-like fluid found in the mouth.

Sanitary Napkin An object made of absorbent material used externally to soak up menstrual blood.

Sapphic Derived from the ancient Greek poetess Sappho who lived on the island of Lesbos and wrote love poems to women. Literary term relating to lesbians.

Satyrist Men who are supposedly sexually insatiable.

Scat Slang term for sexual interest in feces.

Screw Slang for coitus.

Scrotum A pouch of skin and tissue that holds the testicles.

Located just below the penis.

Scum Slang term for ejaculate.

Scum Bag See condom.

Semen Male ejaculate. Slang terms include cum and jism.

Seminal Vesicles A male gland that produces part of the ejaculate (semen).

Sensate Focus A set of exercises adopted from sex therapy to enhance sexual enjoyment and sensuality.

Sensuality The quality of enjoying any stroking or other stimulation which is not overtly sexual.

Seronegative The lack of antibodies to HIV in blood, given as a result of an AIDS antibody test.

Seropositive The presence of antibodies to HIV in blood, given as a result of an AIDS antibody test.

Seroprevalence The number of people who are seropositive.

Serum A component of blood.

Sex General term for erotic activity. Also a reference to gender, i.e. the female sex.

Sex Toys Any object used during sexual activity to enhance sensuality or sexual experience.

Sexual Pleasure A feeling of happiness, delight or satisfaction of the senses relating to sex.

Sexually Transmitted Disease Any disease that can be passed to a sexual partner during a sexual act.

Sexology The scientific study of sex.

Shit Slang term for feces.

Shoot To Slang term for ejaculation.

Simian Retrovirus A form of AIDS found in monkeys and apes. Does not effect humans.

Sixty-nine Slang term for mutual oral sex.

Skin See Condom.

Slave A slang term for a type of masochist.

Slit Slang term for vulva. Often pejorative.

Slut Pejorative term for a person, usually female, who has sex indiscriminately.

Snatch Slang term for vulva.

Social Diseases See Sexually Transmitted Diseases.

Social Kiss See Dry Kiss.

Sodomy Sexual acts involving oral-genital, anal-oral or anal-genital contact.

Soixante-neuf Slang term for mutual oral sex.

Soul Kiss See Wet Kiss.

Speculum A device used by physicians to spread the walls of the vagina to facilitate an examination.

Sperm The male sex cell that combines with the egg in the process of conception. A component of semen.

Sphincter A ring-shaped muscle that surrounds a natural opening in the body and can open or close by expanding or contracting.

Spit Slang term for saliva.

SRV See Simian Retrovirus.

STD(s) See Sexually Transmitted Disease(s).

Street Walker Slang term for prostitute.

Stud Slang term for a virile man, or one who has sex with many partners.

Swing Party Stylized party where participants may engage in sexual acts. Swing parties are usually heterosexual but lesbian activities regularly occur.

Swinger Person who engages in sex at swing parties.

Syphilis A sexually transmitted disease.

Tampon A object made of absorbent material used in the vagina to soak up menstrual blood.

T-cells A type of blood cell that is invaded by HIV.

Teats See Breast.

Testicles Sex glands found in the male which produce both sperm and testosterone. Located in the scrotum. Slang terms include balls, family jewels, gonads, nuts, and orchids.

Testosterone The male sex hormone, found in both men and women.

Thrush See Candidiasis.

Tits See Breasts.

Tramp Pejorative slang term for a woman who supposedly has many sex partners.

Transsexual A person who believes they are really a member of the opposite sex.

Transvestite A man who obtains erotic enjoyment from dressing in women's clothes.

Tribadism A sexual act between two women involving robbing their bodies together. Also used as a synonym for lesbianism.

Trichomonas One-celled organisms that cause vaginal infections.

TS Slang term for transsexual.

TV Slang term for transvestite.

Tumescence The process of getting an erection.

Turd Slang term for feces.

Turned On Slang for sexually excited.

Twat Slang term for vulva or vagina.

Umbilicus Structure that connects the fetus to the placenta.

Urethra The tube that conducts the urine from the bladder out of the body.

Urine A yellow excretory fluid. Unless suffering from an infection, this fluid is sterile and non-toxic.

Urolagnia Another term for urophilia.

Urophilia Erotic attraction to urine, being urinated upon or urinating upon the partner.

Uterus The female organ the lining of which is excreted during the menstrual period. This is a possible site of infection.

Vaccine A substance that causes immunity to a disease.

Vagina A canal in females that leads from the vulva to the uterus Slang terms include box, cunt, quiff, quim, and manhole.

Vaginal-manual intercourse A sexual act involving placing a portion of or the entire hand in a partner's vagina. Can include fisting.

Vas Deferens The tube that transfers sperm from the scrotum to the seminal vesicles.

Vasectomy The severing of the vas deferens. Used as a method to prevent conception.

VD Venereal diseases. See Sexually Transmitted Diseases.

Venereal Diseases See Sexually Transmitted Diseases.

Versatile See Bisexual.

Voyeur Someone who obtains erotic enjoyment from watching another person either naked or engaging in sexual acts.

Vulva Female external genitalia.

Wasserman Test A test for syphilis.

Water Sports Any sexual act involving urine.

Western Blot A test for the presence of the AIDS antibody in blood. More accurate than the ELISA Test, but more expensive.

Wet Dream See Nocturnal Emission.

Wet Kiss A kiss in which both partners open their mouths and stick their tongues in each other's mouth. Exchange of saliva is likely. Also called a French kiss.

Whack Off Slang term for masturbation.
Whore See Prostitute.
Weenie Slang term for penis.
Wife Swapper An older term for a swinger.
Womb See Uterus.
Working Girl See Prostitute.
Zoophilia See Bestiality.

BIBLIOGRAPHY

Aegis. (1998). Procept Presents Findings On Topical Microbicide At 12th World AIDS Conference; In Vitro and In Vivo Experiments Suggest That PRO 2000 Gel Could Protect Against a Variety of Sexually Transmitted Diseases. Retrieved January 22, 2003 from AIDS Education Global Information System website http://www.aegis.com/default.asp?req=http://www.aegis.com/news/bw/1998/BW980701.html

AIDS.ORG Inc. (2002) *Post-Exposure Prophylaxis.* Retrieved February 2, 2003 from AIDS.ORG.Inc. **http://www.aids.org/FactSheets/154-pep.html**

Alexander, N.J. (1996) Barriers to sexually transmitted diseases. *Scientific American Science and Medicine* March/April 1996;3:32-41.

ASHA. (2001). Retrieved December 14, 2002 from American Social Health Association website http://www.ashastd.org/stdfaqs/chancroid.html

ASHA. (2001). Retrieved December 14, 2002 from American Social Health Association website http://www.ashastd.org/stdfaqs/chlamydia.html

ASHA. (2001). Retrieved December 14, 2002 from American Social Health Association website http://www.ashastd.org/stdfaqs/trich.html

ASHA. (2001). Retrieved December 14, 2002 from American Social Health Association website http://www.ashastd.org/stdfaqs/ngu.html

CDC. (1993). *Recommendations for the prevention and management of Chlamydia trachomatis infections*, 1993. *MMWR*; 42 (No. RR-12). Retrieved December 14, 2002 from Centers for Disease Control and Prevention http://www.cdc.gov/mmwr/preview/mmwrhtml/00021622.htm

CDC. (1996). "Update: mortality attributable to HIV infection among persons aged 25-44: United States. *MMWR* 1996;45:121-125. 8

CDC. (1997). *Comprehensive HIV Prevention Messages for Young People.* Retrieved on December 21, 2002 from Centers for Disease Control and Prevention http://www.cdc.gov/nchstp/od/news/compyout.htm

CDC. (1999). *The National Plan to Eliminate Syphilis from the United States.* Retrieved December 26, 2002 from Centers for Disease Control and Prevention website http://www.cdc.gov/stopsyphilis/ExecSumPlan.htm

CDC. (1999). Centers for Disease Control and Prevention *Resurgent bacterial sexually transmitted disease among men who have sex with men – King County, Washington, 1997-1999. MMWR*; 48:773-777. Retrieved December 26, 2002 from Centers for Disease Control and Prevention website http://www.cdc.gov/mmwr/preview/mmwrhtml/mm4835a1.htm

CDC. (2000). *Gonorrhea – United States, 1998. MMWR*;49: 538-42. Retrieved December 26, 2002 from Centers for Disease Control and Prevention website http://www.cdc.gov/epo/mmwr/preview/mmwrhtml/mm4924a5.htm

CDC. (2001). *Outbreak of syphilis among men who have sex with men - Southern California, 2000.MMWR*; 50(7): 117-20. Retrieved on December 21, 2002 from Centers for Disease Control and Prevention http://www.cdc.gov/mmwr/preview/mmwrhtml/mm5007a2.htm

CDC. (2001) STD's in Adolescents and Young Adults. Retrieved January 25, 2003 from the Center for

Disease Control website http://www.cdc.gov/std/stats/TOC2001.htm

CDC. (2001) STD's in Women and Infants. Retrieved January 25, 2003 from the Center for Disease Control website http://www.cdc.gov/std/stats/TOC2001.htm

CDC. (2002). *Male Latex Condoms and Sexually Transmitted Diseases.* Retrieved on December 21, 2002 from Centers for Disease Control and Prevention http://www.cdc.gov/hiv/pubs/faq/faq23.htm

CDC. (2002). *HIV/AIDS Prevention.* Retrieved January 2, 2003 from Centers for Disease Control and Prevention http://www.cdc.gov/hiv/stats.htm

CDC. (2002). *STD Surveillance 2001, Syphilis National Profile.* Retrieved December 22, 2002 from Centers for Disease Control and Prevention http://www.cdc.gov/std/stats/TOC2001.htm

CDC. (2002). *STD Surveillance 2001, STD's in Adolescents and Young Adults Special Focus Profiles* Retrieved December 22, 2002 from Center for Disease Control and Prevention http://www.cdc.gov/std/stats/TOC2001.htm

CDC. (2002). *STD Surveillance 2001 National Profile Gonorrhea.* Retrieved December 22, 2002 from Centers for Disease Control and Prevention http://www.cdc.gov/std/stats/TOC2001.htm

Chun, Rene. (1998). The Goo that Saved the World. *Esquire.* 129-1 p80.

Clincial Trials. (2003). Effects of BufferGel and Pro 2000/5 Gel in Men. Retrieved January 25, 2003 from Clinical Trials website http://www.clinicaltrials.gov/ct/gui/show/NCT00016536;jsessionid=C23774CD9A00B6B9F7C3368EF2D64779?order=2

Cohen MS, Hoffman IF, Royce RA, et al. (1997). Reduction of concentration of HIV-1 in semen after treatment of urethritis: implications for prevention of sexual transmission of HIV-1. *Lancet* 1997;349:1868-73.

Weber, JN (1999). PRO 2000 Gel, A Candidate Topical Microbicide, Can Inhibit Vaginal Simian/Human Immunodeficiency Virus Infection in Rhesus Macaques. Retrieved January 20, 2003 from Center for Disease Control www.cdc.gov/hiv/conferences/hiv99/abstracts/650.pdf

Dotzel, M. M. (2002).. Over-the-Counter Vaginal Contraceptive Drug Products Containing Nonoxynol 9; Required Labeling FR Doc. 03-902 Filed 1-15-03. Retrieved January 26, 2003 from Department of Health and Human Services/Food and Drug Administration http://a257.g.akamaitech.net/7/257/2422/14mar20010800/edocket.access.gpo.gov/2003/03-902.htm

Economist. (2002). Free to Choose. 00130613, 3/2/2002Vol. 362, Issue 8262

Gayle, H.D. (2000). *HIV/AIDS Prevention.* Retrieved on December 22, 2002 from Centers for Disease Control and Prevention website **http://www.cdc.gov/hiv/pubs/mmwr/mmwr11aug00.htm**

HPTN (2003). HPTN 050 Phase 1 Safety and Acceptability Study of the Vaginal Microbicide Agent PMPA Gel. Retrieved January 24, 2003 from HIV Prevention Trials Network website http://www.hptn.org/research_studies/study_details.asp?Protocol+%23=HPTN+050

Key, Keith K., et al. (1996). Distributiona agreement signed for Protectaid in Hong Kong and Macau. *AIDS Weekly*

Plus. 12/16/1996. p16.

Key, Sandra W. et al. (1998). Is Erogel a Miracle Substance for HIV? *AIDS Weekly Plus.* 2/2/1998. p9.

NIAID. (2001). *Human papillomavirus and Genital Warts.* Retrieved January 2, 2003 from National Institute of Allergy and Infectious Diseases http://www.niaid.nih.gov/factsheets/stdhpv.htm

NIAID (2002). NIAID Evaluates N-9 Film as Microbicide. Retrieved January 25, 2003 from Natiional Institute of Allergy and Infectious Diseases (NIAID) website http://www.niaid.nih.gov/publications/agenda/1097/page6.htm

Reich, Wilhelm. (1945). The Sexual Revolution. Farrah, Straus and Giroux. New York Revised 1969.

RHTP (2001-02) Microbicide Develoment. Retrieved January 26, 2003 from Reproductive Health Technologies Project website http://www.rhtp.org/micro/micro_development.htm

ReProtect. (2002). BufferGel. Retrieved January 25, 2003 from ReProtect website http://www.reprotect.com/products.shtml

Staube, Gottfried. (2002). *The Female Condom.* Retrieved December 22, 2002 from http://www.safesex.com

Vogel, Susan E. (1999). NIAID and CC HIV Program. *HIV testing.* Retrieved from http://www.niaid.nih.gov/dir/labs/lir/hiv/packet1.htm on January 2, 2003.

INDEX

A

abdominal breathing 74
abstinence ix
Adult Industry Medical Health Care Foundation (AIM) 11
Age of condoms 51
AIDS 6
AIM 11, 42
Antibody Testing 10
Aquired Immune Deficiency Syndrome 6
Asking for Help 62

B

Basics for Risk Reduction 27
Basic Sexual Rights xii
Bathing with your Partner 97
Beliefs about Sexuality 69
Beliefs about Sex and Pleasure 70
blood 5
blood transfusion 26
blood transfusions 7
body fluids 5
Body Mapping 98
breast feeding 7
BufferGel 46

C

candidiasis (yeast) 7
Carraguard 45
Chemoprophylaxis (Universal Prophylaxis) 37
CHLAMYDIA 14
Cofactors 6
Communicating about Protection 89
Communication Exercise 91
Condoms 48
Contraceptive Sponge 60

O

P

R

S